Sleep Disorders in Selected Psychiatric Settings

Imran S. Khawaja · Thomas D. Hurwitz
Editors

Sleep Disorders in Selected Psychiatric Settings

A Clinical Casebook

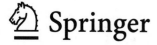 Springer

Editors
Imran S. Khawaja
MD TruCare PA
Grapevine, TX
USA

The University of Oklahoma
OK, USA

Thomas D. Hurwitz
Minneapolis VA Health Care System
Hennepin County Medical Center
University of Minnesota Medical School
Minneapolis, MN
USA

ISBN 978-3-030-59311-7   ISBN 978-3-030-59309-4   (eBook)
https://doi.org/10.1007/978-3-030-59309-4

This Springer imprint is published by the registered company Springer Nature Switzerland AG
The registered company address is: Gewerbestrasse 11, 6330 Cham, Switzerland

Preface

Sleep problems and psychiatric illness go hand in hand. There is no psychiatric disorder during which sleep is not disturbed, and there has been an increasing emphasis on recognizing and treating sleep disorders in patients with comorbid psychiatric illness. Evidence supports a bidirectional relationship between the two domains. Because of this relationship, increasing clinical sensitivity to sleep disturbance enhances the monitoring of severity, natural history, the progress of therapy, and the risk of relapse of psychiatric disorders. Clinicians must become increasingly familiar with these issues. For instance, we now recognize insomnia as a symptom of mood disorder and a predictor of its occurrence, relapse, and severity. We are learning that sleep-disordered breathing is frequently co-morbid with depression.

In our first book, *Comorbid Sleep and Psychiatric Disorders: A Clinical Case Book*, 23 cases are presented to highlight this relationship. This was intended to help busy clinicians learn about how to approach these issues more effectively.

In this second volume, we provide 19 additional cases to supplement what was introduced initially. These include various examples of insomnia and substance-induced sleep disorders as well as specialized areas of interest that cover women and children and sleep difficulties in inpatient settings.

Though several textbooks on sleep disorders are available for psychiatrists, we hope that a practically oriented casebook can provide trainees and experienced providers with a useful guide to assist in their clinical practice.

Most of these examples represent common occurrences, though some may seem unusual. We hope they will stimulate further study and increase familiarity.

We have made an effort to keep these chapters brief and easily digestible.

Questions are posed to stimulate the reader, followed by a discussion of diagnosis, treatment, and useful take-home points. We hope that this book will inform and stimulate clinicians from various backgrounds.

Grapevine, TX, USA
Minneapolis, MN, USA

Imran S. Khawaja
Thomas D. Hurwitz

Contents

Contributors

Noha Abdel-Gawad Inova Fairfax Hospital, Department of Psychiatry, Falls Church, VA, USA

Adam S. Akers Department of Internal Medicine, Sidra Medicine, Doha, Qatar

Melissa Allen UT Health Harris County Psychiatric Center, Department of Psychiatry and Behavioral Sciences, Houston, TX, USA

Sophia Banu Menninger Department of Psychiatry & Behavioral Sciences, Baylor College of Medicine, Ben Taub Hospital Center, Department of Psychiatry, Houston, TX, USA

Irina Baranskaya University of Oklahoma Health Sciences Center, Department of Psychiatry and Behavioral Sciences, Oklahoma City, OK, USA

Todd M. Bishop VISN 2 Center of Excellence for Suicide Prevention (COE), Department of Veterans Affairs, Canandaigua, NY, USA

Gregory S. Carter UT Southwestern Sleep Medicine Fellowship Program, Department of Neurology and Neurotherapeutics at The University of Texas Southwestern Medical Center at Dallas, Dallas, TX, USA

Teresa Chan-Leveno University of Texas Southwestern Medical Center, Department of Otolaryngology, Dallas, TX, USA

Christopher T. Copeland The University of Oklahoma, College of Medicine, Department of Psychiatry & Behavioral Sciences, Neuropsychology Lab, Oklahoma City, OK, USA

Neelam Danish Cardiovascular Surgery, UT Southwestern Medical Center, Dallas, TX, USA

Patricia Dickmann Mental Health, Minneapolis VA Medical Center, Minneapolis, MN, USA

Aimee T. Dunnam The University of Texas Arlington, Arlington, TX, USA

Ayesha Ebrahim Endocrinology, MD TruCare PA, Grapevine, TX, USA

Omo Edaki Department of Psychiatry Clinical Research, John Peter Smith Hospital, Fort Worth, TX, USA

Vijaya Bharathi Ekambaram Touro University California, Vallejo, California, USA

Bita Farhadpour Dignity Health, Houston, TX, USA

Yasmin Gharbaoui University of Texas Health Science Center at Houston, Department of Psychiatry, Houston, TX, USA

Morgan B. Glusman The University of Oklahoma, College of Medicine, Department of Psychiatry & Behavioral Sciences, Neuropsychology Lab, Oklahoma City, OK, USA

Mollie Gordon Ben Taub Hospital, Menninger Department of Psychiatry and Behavioral Sciences, Bellaire, TX, USA

Ani Gupta The Ohio State Wexner Medical Center, Department of Neurology, Columbus, OH, USA

Aaron B. Holley Walter Reed National Military Medical Center, Department of Pulmonary and Critical Care Medicine, Bethesda, MD, USA

Jessica Holster The University of Oklahoma, College of Medicine, Department of Psychiatry & Behavioral Sciences, Neuropsychology Lab, Oklahoma City, OK, USA

John C. Hunninghake Brooke Army Medical Center, Department of Pulmonary/Critical Care Medicine, JBSA Fort Sam Houston, TX, USA

Conrad Iber Department of Medicine, M Health Fairview, Minneapolis, MN, USA

Bibi Aneesah Jaumally UT Health Science Center at Houston, Department of Internal Medicine, Houston, TX, USA

Safia S. Khan Department of Family and Community Medicine, Department of Neurology and Neurotherapeutics at University of Texas Southwestern Medical Center, Dallas, TX, USA
Parkland Sleep Center, Parkland Medical Hospital, Dallas, TX, USA
Texas Health Resources Presbyterian Hospital, Dallas, TX, USA

Imran S. Khawaja MD TruCare PA, Grapevine, TX, USA
Department of Psychiatry, The University of Oklahoma, OK, USA

Elliott Kyung Lee Royal Ottawa Mental Health Centre Geriatric Psychiatry Program and University of Ottawa Department of Psychiatry, Ottawa, ON, USA
Royal Ottawa Mental Health Centre Sleep Disorders Clinic, Institute for Mental Health Research (IMHR), Ottawa, ON, USA

Won Young Lee University of Texas Southwestern Medical Center, Department of Internal Medicine, Dallas, TX, USA

Jie Luo Sleep Center, Shanghai International Medical Center, Shanghai, China

Shahram Moghadam Michael E. DeBakey VA Medical Center, Department of Medicine, Houston, TX, USA

Nidal Moukaddam Department of Psychiatry and Behavioral Sciences, Baylor College of Medicine, Houston, TX, USA

S. Kamal Naqvi Department of Pediatrics, UT Southwestern Medical Center/ Children's Health, Sleep Disorders Center, Dallas, TX, USA

Michelle Nazario Menninger Department of Psychiatry & Behavioral Sciences - Baylor College of Medicine, Houston, TX, USA

Ben Taub General Hospital, Houston, TX, USA

Edore Onigu-Otite Menninger Department of Psychiatry & Behavioral Sciences - Baylor College of Medicine, Houston, TX, USA

Ben Taub Neuropsychiatry Center, Houston, TX, USA

Britta Klara Ostermeyer University of Oklahoma Health Sciences Center, Department of Psychiatry and Behavioral Sciences, Oklahoma City, OK, USA

Wilfred R. Pigeon VISN 2 Center of Excellence for Suicide Prevention (COE), Department of Veterans Affairs, Canandaigua, NY, USA

Marie-Hélène Rivard Royal Ottawa Mental Health Centre Geriatric Psychiatry Program and University of Ottawa Department of Psychiatry, Ottawa, ON, USA

Mary Rose Baylor College of Medicine, Department of Medicine, Houston, TX, USA

Rachel Rosen Children's Health, Sleep Disorder Center, Dallas, TX, USA

Asim A. Shah Menninger Department of Psychiatry and Behavioral Sciences, Baylor College of Medicine, Houston, TX, USA

Amir Sharafkhaneh Michael E. DeBakey VA Medical Center, Department of Medicine, Houston, TX, USA

Supriya Singh Michael E. DeBakey VA Medical Center, Department of Medicine, Houston, TX, USA

Heather Swanson Addiction Recovery Services, Minneapolis Veterans Affairs Medical Center, Minneapolis, MN, USA

Department of Psychiatry, University of Minnesota, Minneapolis VA Health Care Center, Minneapolis, MN, USA

Mental Health, Minneapolis VA Medical Center, Minneapolis, MN, USA

Stephen Talsness Department of Psychiatry, Minneapolis VA Health Care System, Minneapolis, MN, USA

Natasha Thrower Pediatric and Adolescent Health Center, Pasadena, TX, USA

Menninger Department of Psychiatry & Behavioral Sciences - Baylor College of Medicine, Houston, TX, USA

Alison Uku Department of Obstetrics and Gynecology, Sidra Medicine, Doha, Qatar

Sidarth Wakhlu Department of Psychiatry, UT Southwestern Medical Center, Dallas, TX, USA

Robert J. Walter Brooke Army Medical Center, Department of Pulmonary/Critical Care Medicine, JBSA Fort Sam Houston, TX, USA

Anna Wani UT Southwestern Medical Center/Children's Health, Sleep Disorders Center, Dallas, TX, USA

Felice Watt Department of Psychiatry, Sidra Medicine, Doha, Qatar

Joseph Westermeyer Department of Psychiatry, University of Minnesota, Minneapolis VA Health Care Center, Minneapolis, MN, USA

Charlie Wu Sleep Lab, Shanghai International Medical Center, Shanghai, China

Chester Wu Stanford Health Care, Department of Psychiatry, Redwood City, CA, USA

Adam N. Young Kadena Medical Group/U.S. Navy Hospital Okinawa, Critical Care Air Transport/Intensive Care Unit, APO, AP, Japan

Zakaria Zayour Mental Health, Dallas VA Medical Center, Dallas, TX, USA

Part I

Cases of Insomnia

Benzodiazepine Withdrawal Insomnia

Zakaria Zayour and Sidarth Wakhlu

Benzodiazepine Withdrawal Insomnia

Mrs. K is a 55-year-old Caucasian female with history of anxiety, insomnia, hypothyroidism, and pre-diabetes. She had been on diazepam 5 mg at bedtime for insomnia prescribed by her PCP for the past four years. However, she started misusing her diazepam and was taking more than prescribed for the last two years. In the last year, she was taking between 20 and 30 mg a day of diazepam and was repeatedly asking for early refills. Her primary care physician (PCP) suspected she was abusing her diazepam and informed her he will no longer be able to continue prescribing it for her and that she will need to undergo inpatient detoxification. She declined and instead started doctor shopping for benzodiazepines. By mid-2017, her prescription monitoring program (PMP) record showed that she was receiving prescriptions for multiple benzodiazepines (diazepam, clonazepam, zolpidem, and temazepam) from three different providers. It was not until the patient was arrested and charged with driving under the influence (DUI) that she realized she needed to get help for her addiction.

The patient denied alcohol use and abusing any other prescription pills or illicit substances. She is a nonsmoker.

The patient was admitted to the psychiatric inpatient unit for benzodiazepine detoxification. Her last benzodiazepine (BZD) use was around 48 hours prior to admission. She was reporting rebound anxiety, mild tremors, and anorexia. She complained of significant insomnia and reported sleeping 3–4 hours the previous two nights prior to admission which in turn caused her fatigue and dysphoria.

Z. Zayour (✉)
Mental Health, Dallas VA Medical Center, Dallas, TX, USA
e-mail: Zakaria.zayour@va.gov

S. Wakhlu
Department of Psychiatry, UT Southwestern Medical Center, Dallas, TX, USA

© Springer Nature Switzerland AG 2021
I. S. Khawaja, T. D. Hurwitz (eds.), *Sleep Disorders in Selected Psychiatric Settings*, https://doi.org/10.1007/978-3-030-59309-4_1

The patient denied any previous history of seizures or delirium tremens (DTs) but reported significant anxiety, tremors, and insomnia when she would run out of BZDs for 2–3 days.

Outpatient Medications

Levothyroxine 75 mcg daily, metformin 500 mg bid, diazepam 10 mg bid, clonazepam 1 mg at bedtime, zolpidem 10 mg at bedtime

Vital Signs

T = 37.5 C; BP = 133/72; P = 97; RR = 22; Pain = 0/10

Physical Exam

- No significant findings

Mental Status Exam

The patient was wearing hospital clothes, appeared stated age, and was fairly groomed. She had mild tremors but no abnormal movements otherwise. She had a stable gait and did not show any signs of muscle weakness. She was cooperative with the interviewer. Her speech was intact. Her mood was "anxious" and her affect was congruent with her stated mood. Her thought process was logical, linear, and goal oriented. Her thought content was devoid of suicidal or homicidal ideas or delusions. She did not have any hallucinations. She was alerted and oriented to person, place, time, and situation. She had average intelligence and intact fund of knowledge. Her insight and judgment were fair.

Labs

- CBC, CMP, TSH, and vitamin D are within normal limits.
- Urine drug screen + BZD; BAL <5.

EKG

Normal sinus rhythm (NSR), no abnormal findings, QTc 411

The patient was placed on CIWA-Ar and received a total of 6 mg of lorazepam during the first 24 hours with a high CIWA-Ar score of 10. As for sleep, she was given trazodone 50 mg, melatonin 3 mg, and gabapentin 600 mg. However, she reported that she slept only 3 hours and was getting more irritable and frustrated.

The patient received a total of 4 mg of lorazepam the following 24 hours with a high CIWA-Ar score of 7. Her sleep regimen was increased to trazodone 200 mg, melatonin 3 mg, and gabapentin 900 mg. The next day, the patient reported only a slight improvement in sleep. She was able to complete the detox fairly well, aside from her insomnia, and be discharged home.

On follow-up 1 week later, she continued to report significant insomnia and daytime fatigue. She declined referral to cognitive behavioral therapy for insomnia (CBT-I). The plan was to short trial of quetiapine 100 mg at bedtime for sleep. The patient's sleep started to improve within 1–2 weeks, and she was able to get off the quetiapine on the 4-week follow-up visit.

Diagnosis

Rebound insomnia

Discussion

Although the American Psychiatric Association (APA) and several other authorities caution against the long-term use of benzodiazepines, especially in older patients [1], they are still widely used for the treatment of insomnia as well as anxiety [2]. Clinical guidelines recommend behavioral interventions as the first step in the treatment of insomnia [3] as they have similar efficacy compared to BZDs in the short term [4] and longer-lasting effects after stopping treatment [5]. Moreover, there is very limited evidence that BZDs actually retain their efficacy with long-term treatment [5] while at the same time carrying a significant risk for withdrawal symptoms when abruptly discontinued as well as abuse [6]. Despite this, the number of adults filling a benzodiazepine prescription increased 67%, from 8.1 million to 13.5 million, between 1997 and 2013 [7]. This was associated with a fourfold increase in overdose deaths involving BZDs [7].

Upon discontinuation, rebound insomnia and anxiety are common manifestations of the BZD withdrawal course [8]. Once the medication is reinstituted, those symptoms rapidly resolve which in turn gives patients a false sense of efficacy [8]. BZD rebound insomnia is characterized by increased wakefulness beyond baseline levels following discontinuation of the BZD [9]. It can occur after single, nightly doses of BZD even for short duration [10] and is more likely to occur with BZD of shorter half-lives like triazolam (4.5 hours) as compared to BZD with long half-lives like diazepam (47–100 hours) [11]. Even after brief and intermittent use, short-acting BZD like triazolam produced rebound insomnia after abrupt withdrawal [12], thereby increasing risk for medication misuse and dependence. Hypnotic BZDs can be abused for recreational purposes, i.e., for a "high," or for "quasi-therapeutic" purposes [13].

Our patient was using diazepam to self-treat her insomnia. She is a middle-aged female with no comorbid history of substance use and is less likely to be abusing her medication for recreational purposes. However, regardless of the purpose of BZD abuse/misuse, the first part of treatment is a safe detox program with a significant emphasis on targeting insomnia in order to mitigate the risk of returning to BZD use or of relapse. To avoid using BZD receptor agonists, it is quite common to use medications with an off label indication for insomnia to achieve that goal [14]. Those medications include trazodone, mirtazapine, antiepileptics, and atypical antipsychotics. Some of these medications have a significant adverse effect profile if used in the long run and are more appropriate for acute or short-term use.

It is imperative to be proactive about the treatment of insomnia during and after the detoxification course in order to decrease the risk of returning to BZDs or seeking illicit hypnotics/sedatives for self-treatment. In the outpatient setting, non-pharmacological treatments should then be offered including stimulus control therapy, relaxation training, and CBT-I. Those three modalities are individually effective in the treatment of chronic insomnia [15].

References

1. Salzman C. The APA Task Force report on benzodiazepine dependence, toxicity, and abuse. Am J Psychiatr. 1991;148(2):151–2.
2. Cunningham CM, Hanley GE, Morgan S. Patterns in the use of benzodiazepines in British Columbia: examining the impact of increasing research and guideline cautions against long-term use. Health Policy. 2010;97(2–3):122–9.
3. Morgenthaler TI, et al.; Standards of Practice Committee of the American Academy of Sleep Medicine. Practice parameters for the clinical evaluation and treatment of circadian rhythm sleep disorders: an American Academy of Sleep Medicine report. Sleep. 2007;30(11):1445–59.
4. Smith MT, Perlis ML, Park A, et al. Comparative meta-analysis of pharmacotherapy and behavior therapy for persistent insomnia. Am J Psychiatry. 2002;159(1):5–11.
5. Riemann D, et al. The treatments of chronic insomnia: A review of benzodiazepine receptor agonists and psychological and behavioral therapies. Sleep Med Rev. 2009;13(3):205–14.
6. Fenton MC, Keyes KM, Martins SS, Hasin DS. The role of a prescription in anxiety medication use, abuse, and dependence. Am J Psychiatry. 2010;167(10):1247–53.
7. Bachhuber MA, Hennessy S, Cunningham CO, Starrels JL. Increasing benzodiazepine prescriptions and overdose mortality in the United States, 1996-2013. Am J Public Health. 2016;106(4):686–8. https://doi.org/10.2105/AJPH.2016.303061. Epub 2016 Feb 18.
8. Chouinard G. Issues in the clinical use of benzodiazepines: potency, withdrawal, and rebound. J Clin Psychiatry. 2004;65 Suppl 5:7–12.
9. Roehrs T, Roth T. Hypnotics: an update. Curr Neurol Neurosci Rep. 2003;3(2):181–4.
10. Kales A, Scharf MB, Kales JD. Rebound insomnia: a new clinical syndrome. Science. 1978;201:1039–41.
11. Kales A, Scharf MB, Kales JD, Soldatos CR. Rebound insomnia a potential hazard following withdrawal of certain benzodiazepines. JAMA. 1979;241(16):1692–5. https://doi.org/10.1001/jama.1979.03290420018017.
12. Kales A, et al. Rebound insomnia after only brief and intermittent use of rapidly eliminated benzodiazepines. Clin Pharmacol Ther. 1991;49(4):468–76.

13. Griffiths RR, Johnson MW. Relative abuse liability of hypnotic drugs: a conceptual framework and algorithm for differentiating among compounds. J Clin Psychiatry. 2005;66 Suppl 9:31–41.
14. Lie JD, Tu KN, Shen DD, Wong BM. Pharmacological treatment of insomnia. Pharm Ther. 2015;40(11):759–71.
15. Morgenthaler T, et al. Practice parameters for the psychological and behavioral treatment of insomnia: an update. An American Academy of Sleep Medicine Report Sleep. 2006;29(11):14151419. https://doi.org/10.1093/sleep/29.11.1415.

Case Study: Brief CBT-I and Medication Taper with a Veteran Experiencing Insomnia and Suicidal Ideation

Todd M. Bishop and Wilfred R. Pigeon

Clinical History/Case

Patient X was a 62-year-old, married, Caucasian female. The patient is a veteran of the US army and served on active duty from the mid-1970s until the mid-1990s upon which time she retired from service. Patient X's presenting complaint was that of insomnia characterized by a series of awakenings during the night and a prominent early awakening each morning. Sleep onset latency, which averaged 11.4 minutes in the week prior to treatment, was likely historically suppressed via the patient's longtime use of temazepam, which she estimated she had been using for approximately 10 years. The patient also endorsed suffering from comorbid medical conditions which interfered with her sleep including depression, migraine headaches, and chronic back pain.

Chronic back pain, preexisting mental illness (depression), and a history of sexual trauma were among the factors that *predisposed* the patient to the development of insomnia disorder. At the initiation of treatment, however, the insomnia disorder had been present for several years, and it was unclear what *precipitated* its onset. Many factors served to *perpetuate* Patient X's insomnia, including poor sleep hygiene, a variable rise time, unmanaged chronic back pain, and sleep-interfering cognitions. Sleep-interfering behaviors included the following: (a) having different bed and rise times than her spouse, (b) her spouse watching TV in bed, (c) having a different preferred temperature for the bedroom than her spouse, and (d) having several dogs share the bedroom.

T. M. Bishop (✉) · W. R. Pigeon
VISN 2 Center of Excellence for Suicide Prevention (COE), Department of Veterans Affairs, Canandaigua, NY, USA

Department of Psychiatry, University of Rochester Medical Center, Rochester, NY, USA
e-mail: todd.bishop@va.gov

© Springer Nature Switzerland AG 2021
I. S. Khawaja, T. D. Hurwitz (eds.), *Sleep Disorders in Selected Psychiatric Settings*, https://doi.org/10.1007/978-3-030-59309-4_2

Patient X reported experiencing depression for much of her life. She had pursued psychotherapy to address her depression for several years and continued to do so throughout the current treatment episode. In addition, the patient reported that she had attempted suicide once at the age of 18. The suicide attempt was made by ingesting sleeping pills and resulted in hospitalization. Patient X also endorsed current suicidal ideation at the onset of treatment. She described active thoughts of suicide that occurred daily and felt persistent or nearly continuous. However, she denied the presence of a plan of how she would end her life as well as any intention to act on these thoughts. The patient also believed that she was able to control these thoughts and was able to identify deterrents kept her from acting on her ideations.

Pharmacologic Interventions

For several years prior to this treatment episode, Patient X had been prescribed quetiapine fumarate 150 mg at bed for mood, fluoxetine 40 mg for depression, and temazepam 15 mg at bed for sleep. The patient also used excedrin over the counter to manage migraine headaches. Five months prior to the current treatment episode, Patient X's psychiatrist replaced the temazepam with diazepam and began a taper regimen that ended in October of 2015, 1 month before the patient initiated CBT-I. It would seem that the taper from temazepam was particularly prudent as the Food and Drug Administration has cautioned its use among individuals experiencing severe depression or suicidal ideation [1], both of which Patient X endorsed.

As the temazepam lost its effectiveness, the patient began to supplement with melatonin. In the course of the 12 months prior to treatment, Patient X had increased her use of over-the-counter melatonin to 40 mg per evening, an alarming 20 times the common dose of 2 mg. It should be noted that the American Academy of Sleep Medicine suggests that clinicians not use melatonin as a treatment for sleep onset or sleep maintenance insomnia [2].

Treatment Episode

Cognitive Behavioral Therapy for Insomnia

The patient came under author TB's care (supervised by author WP) during the course of research examining the efficacy of brief cognitive behavioral therapy for insomnia (CBT-I). As part of this protocol, the patient underwent pre- and post-treatment batteries of measures and completed four sessions of CBT-I. Sessions occurred between November and December 2015. In addition, the patient's current level of suicidal ideation and safety were assessed at each session. Although Patient X did not require it to be enacted, a robust safety protocol including clinical backup and safety planning was in place.

Special Studies

While in treatment, Patient X kept a sleep diary each morning upon awakening and provided a completed diary to the therapist at the start of each session. For the purposes of this chapter, we report on sleep onset latency (SL), time awake after sleep onset (WASO), total sleep time (TST), and sleep efficiency (SE; TST divided by time in bed x 100%). In addition, the patient completed the Insomnia Severity Index [3, 4] (ISI) and Patient Health Questionnaire (PHQ-9) prior to each therapy session. Two additional measures, the Multidimensional Pain Inventory [5] (MPI) and the Columbia-Suicide Severity Rating Scale [6] (C-SSRS),were included in the pre-and post-treatment assessment packet.

Session One

Session one consisted of psychoeducation regarding sleep and the development of insomnia as well as the introduction of stimulus control and sleep restriction. Patient X's sleep diary data revealed an average sleep onset latency of 11.4 minutes, a WASO of 43.6 minutes, and 454.3 minutes of TST (see Fig. 2.1). When asked to describe her pre-bedtime regimen, she reported highly variable bed (~11:30 pm) and wake (~7:30 am) times. In the hours leading up to sleep, the patient watched

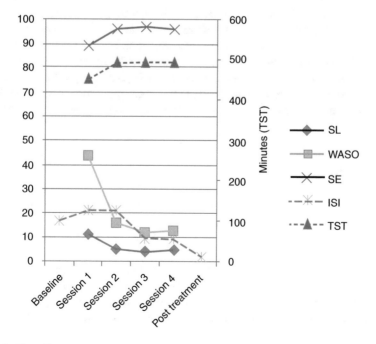

Fig. 2.1 Sleep diary outcomes

television and often dosed on the couch. Her husband would go to bed at 8 pm and rise at 430 am for work each morning, which would interfere with her ability to maintain sleep and contribute to early morning awakenings. The patient stated that she took 40 mg of melatonin at 8 pm each night and that she would begin to feel drowsy around 9 pm, but not enter bed until much later. The patient endorsed a willingness to decrease the dose of melatonin, and we agreed to start a taper the following week. Sleep was restricted to 7.5 hours, and regular bed (12:00 am) and wake (7:30 am) times were established. In regard to the sleep environment, we were able to identify two between session goals including (1) removing the collars from the pets prior to getting into bed and (2) leaving the bed after 15 minutes of sleeplessness.

Session Two

At the beginning of session 2, the patient reported that she was largely compliant with the recommended changes to her sleep environment and was able to consistently keep to her prescribed wake time. She did, however, report having difficulty staying awake until her prescribed bedtime (12:00 am) as her granddaughter was visiting this week and the patient was more tired than is typical for her. She also stated that she felt that 7 am was a more natural wake time for her. We ultimately decided on shifting her sleep window to 11 pm to 7 am. Patient X was also able to identify her caffeine and nicotine consumption (three-fourths pack of cigarettes per day) as additional behaviors that interfere with her sleep. She ultimately decided to switch to decaffeinated coffee in the afternoons and smoke her last cigarette at least 30 minutes prior to initiating sleep. We also agreed to begin a gradual reduction in the use of the over-the-counter melatonin from 40 to 20 mg per evening. As part of session two, the patient also designed a more stable, relaxing pre-bedtime routine. Patient X decided on brushing her teeth, taking some quiet time to sit on her porch away from the television, praying, and taking a warm shower to help with her back pain.

Session Three

As can be seen in Fig. 2.1, by session three, the patient began to see improvements in SL, which had decreased to approximately 4 minutes, a 27% reduction in WASO, and an increase in SE from 89% to 97%. We held the sleep window steady at 11 pm to 7 am and focused on being consistent about bed and wake times. The patient reported that she had successfully switched to decaffeinated coffee and that she was able to practice most elements of her new pre-bedtime routine most nights. We further reduced the dose of melatonin from 20 to 10 mg per evening. At this time, a marked decrease in depression also was noted on the PHQ-9 (see Fig. 2.2).

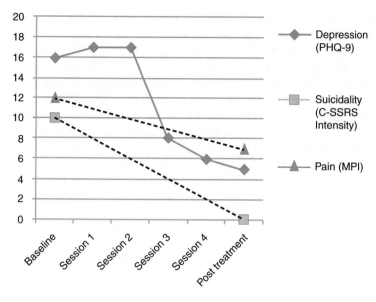

Fig. 2.2 Treatment effects: psychopathology

Session Four

The fourth and final session followed what Patient X described as a high stress period consisting of the holidays, visiting family, and a scheduled surgery for a family member. Patient X's sleep diaries revealed that she was able to maintain her improvements in SL, WASO, and SE. In this final session, we recapped what had been learned in sessions one through three as well as discussed relapse prevention. This included a discussion of the potential for rebound insomnia and the exploration of cognitive reframing such as conceptualizing "one bad night of sleep as just one bad night." Patient agreed to continue keeping sleep diary for several weeks post treatment in order to solidify her treatment gains. She also requested that her bedtime be moved back to 10:30 pm allowing her a sleep window of 8.5 hours. We further reduced the dose of melatonin to 5 mg. Patient stated that she intended to discontinue the use of melatonin in the weeks following treatment.

Results

Post-treatment

Patient X was largely adherent to the prescribed interventions and was invested in her treatment. In regard to Patient X's sleep, over the course of the treatment episode, increases in SE and TST, as well as corresponding decreases in SL, WASO, and ISI severity score, were observed (see Fig. 2.1). These improvements in sleep parameters were anticipated given the demonstrated efficacy of CBT-I [7, 8]. This case, however, presented challenges that had the potential to reduce the effectiveness of CBT-I such as (a) delivery of four as opposed to the standard six to eight sessions of CBT-I, (b) the recent tapering of Temazepam and Diazepam, (c) the gradual dose reduction of melatonin, and (d) psychiatric comorbidities.

In addition to improved sleep, the patient reported clinically significant reductions in chronic pain, depression, and suicidal ideation (see Fig. 2.2). Over the course of treatment, depression scores on the PHQ-9 dropped from 16 (moderately severe depression) to 5 (mild depression). Suicidal ideation, which at the outset of treatment was reported to be persistent and occur daily, was absent at follow-up. As the melatonin taper and CBT-I occurred concurrently, we are unable to conclusively attribute the origin of the marked reduction in psychopathology. However, the current literature does not suggest a link between melatonin and suicidality. Thus, it is more likely that reductions in depression and suicidal ideation were the product of improved sleep and hypothesized mechanisms of action (e.g., improved feelings of self-efficacy, improved executive functioning and ability to utilize coping strategies).

Follow-Up

Patient X continued to receive care through the Veterans Health Administration following the completion of CBT-I in December 2015. In the same month that she finished CBT-I, and with her depressive symptoms reduced, her psychiatrist began a gradual dose reduction of the quetiapine fumarate with a taper being completed 2 months later in February 2016. Patient X continued to use 3 mg of melatonin in the months following CBT-I but ceased using the hormone as of September 2016. Seven months after treatment, in July 2016, the patient was started on topiramate 200 mg bid for migraine prevention.

In December 2016, a full year following the course of CBT-I, the patient again began to report sleep onset insomnia that was precipitated by family stress and the death of a close friend. The treating psychiatrist referenced back to the completed CBT-I treatment episode and also suggested changes in sleep hygiene. The patient, being somewhat resistant to engage the recommended behaviors, was started on a course of trazodone 50 mg qd which has been ongoing for 9 months. Notably, there has not been a recurrence of the suicidal thought observed at the start of the treatment episode, and the reductions in depressive symptomatology following CBT-I have held and are being successfully managed with fluoxetine and individual psychotherapy. The patient continues to regularly engage in care and has even attempted a smoking cessation protocol in the past year.

Differential Diagnosis and Diagnosis

The patient did not report symptoms consistent with other sleep disorders that may be contributing to her sleep complaint (e.g., narcolepsy, sleep apnea, restless legs syndrome, nightmare disorder, parasomnias). For instance, the patient denied snoring, falling asleep at inappropriate places, being told she stops breathing when asleep, or other symptoms suggestive of obstructive sleep apnea. Feelings of discomfort or restlessness in the bed were best attributed to back pain and did not appear to indicate restless legs syndrome or periodic limb movements of sleep symptoms. Patient X also denied symptoms of narcolepsy (e.g., cataplexy, sleep paralysis) or presence of nightmares. In addition, although her sleep schedule is varied and she may go to bed late, she does not present with a sleep pattern suggestive of a circadian rhythm disorder. Nocturnal events associated with parasomnias are also denied. The patient sleep complaints are most consistent, therefore, with a diagnosis of insomnia disorder. In addition, neither her depression nor pain condition appears to have been a sole contributor to the development of insomnia, although they were at the time of evaluation possibly contributing to the severity of insomnia.

- Major depressive disorder, recurrent, moderate (F33.1)
- Insomnia disorder (F51.01)
- Back pain (M54.5)

General Remarks

Insomnia, whether a co-occurring disorder or the symptom of an underlying behavioral health condition, warrants early attention in the course of treatment. Insomnia has been demonstrated to precipitate new onset mental illness [9] and blunt response to treatments aimed at addressing depression [10] and has been associated with increased risk for suicide [11, 12]. Thus, it is important to consider insomnia's role in the course and development of patients' psychopathology and to address it accordingly. The present case highlights the importance of asking about patients' over-the-counter medications and substances (e.g., melatonin, energy drinks) that may affect sleep or the symptoms that may mimic or exacerbate those of a mental health disorder (e.g., excessive caffeine increasing irritability). Behavioral interventions for insomnia can be successfully delivered in the context of co-occurring psychopathology.

Pearls/Take-Home Points
- Insomnia may be addressed in the context of several common medical and psychiatric conditions; this case demonstrates how CBT for insomnia may even be delivered when a patient is experiencing suicidal ideation when a sound plan for assessing and managing safety is in place.
- Behavioral interventions for insomnia may be delivered effectively in conjunction with a medication taper.
- Providers should continue to conduct thorough assessments regarding patients' medication regimens including inquiries regarding the names and doses of over-the-counter medications that the patient may be using.

References

1. Restoril [package insert]. Hazelwood: Mallinckrodt Inc; 2016.
2. Sateia MJ, Buysse DJ, Krystal AD, Neubauer DN, Heald JL. Clinical practice guideline for the pharmacologic treatment of chronic insomnia in adults: an American Academy of Sleep Medicine clinical practice guideline. J Clin Sleep Med. 2017;13(2):307–49.
3. Bastien CH, Vallieres A, Morin CM. Validation of the Insomnia Severity Index as an outcome measure for insomnia research. Sleep Med. 2001;2(4):297–307.
4. Morin CM. Insomnia: psychological assessment and management. New York: Guilford Press; 1993.
5. Kerns RD, Turk DC, Rudy TE. The West Haven-Yale Multidimensional Pain Inventory (WHYMPI). Pain. 1985;23(4):345–56.
6. Posner K, Brown GK, Stanley B, et al. The Columbia-suicide severity rating scale: initial validity and internal consistency findings from three multisite studies with adolescents and adults. Am J Psychiatry. 2011;168(12):1266–77.
7. Irwin MR, Cole JC, Nicassio PM. Comparative meta-analysis of behavioral interventions for insomnia and their efficacy in middle-aged adults and in older adults 55+ years of age. Health Psychol. 2006;25(1):3–14.
8. Pigeon WR, Bishop TM, Marcus J. Current pharmacological and nonpharmacological options for the management of insomnia. Clin Med Insights Ther. 2013;5:151–62.
9. Pigeon WR, Bishop TM, Krueger KM. Insomnia as a precipitating factor in new onset mental illness: a systematic review of recent findings. Curr Psychiatry Rep. 2017;19(8):44.
10. Baglioni C, Spiegelhalder K, Nissen C, Riemann D. Clinical implications of the causal relationship between insomnia and depression: how individually tailored treatment of sleeping difficulties could prevent the onset of depression. EPMA J. 2011;2(3):287–93.
11. Pigeon WR, Pinquart M, Conner K. Meta-analysis of sleep disturbance and suicidal thoughts and behaviors. J Clin Psychiatry. 2012;73(9):1160–7.
12. Pigeon WR, Bishop TM, Titus CE. The relationship of sleep disturbance to suicidal ideation, suicide attempts and suicide among adults: a systematic review. Psychiatr Ann. 2016;46(3):177–86.

Suggested Reading

Bernert RA, Joiner TE, Cukrowicz KC, Schmidt NB, Krakow B. Suicidality and sleep disturbance. Sleep. 2005;28(9):1135–41.

Pigeon WR, Pinquart M, Conner K. Meta-analysis of sleep disturbance and suicidal thoughts and behaviors. J Clin Psychiatry. 2012;73(9):e1160–7.

Sateia MJ, Buysse DJ, Krystal AD, Neubauer DN, Heald JL. Clinical practice guideline for the pharmacologic treatment of chronic insomnia in adults: an American Academy of Sleep Medicine clinical practice guideline. J Clin Sleep Med. 2017;13(2):307–49.

Part II

Substances and Sleep

Some Say Marijuana Helps with Sleep. Is It True?

3

Aimee T. Dunnam, Jie Luo, Charlie Wu, and Imran S. Khawaja

Clinical History

Mrs. X is a 58-year-old Caucasian female with a diagnosis of bipolar I disorder, generalized anxiety disorder, insomnia (unspecified), chronic pain syndrome, migraine headaches (uncomplicated), and cannabis dependence. She was diagnosed with bipolar I disorder when she was in her 30s but was unmanaged for significant periods in her life, and even at present, she denies she has bipolar disorder. Per the patient's report, she has unmanaged anxiety and insomnia, depression, pain, and headaches. She has also trialed many different combinations of medications to manage symptoms of her bipolar disorder, with varying degrees of success. The patient had tried anxiolytics and has a history of long-term benzodiazepine (clonazepam) use until 4 months ago when she was admitted to an inpatient psychiatric facility to undergo a managed withdrawal. She was on clonazepam for 3 years prior to her facilitated withdrawal.

The patient presents with complaints of anxiety, restlessness, paranoia, and insomnia. She states that daily cannabis appears to no longer be as effective as previously in managing her anxiety and sleeplessness. She reports smoking at

A. T. Dunnam (✉)
The University of Texas Arlington, Arlington, TX, USA

J. Luo
Sleep Center, Shanghai International Medical Center, Shanghai, China

C. Wu
Sleep Lab, Shanghai International Medical Center, Shanghai, China

I. S. Khawaja
MD TruCare PA, Grapevine, TX, USA

Department of Psychiatry, The University of Oklahoma, OK, USA

© Springer Nature Switzerland AG 2021
I. S. Khawaja, T. D. Hurwitz (eds.), *Sleep Disorders in Selected Psychiatric Settings*, https://doi.org/10.1007/978-3-030-59309-4_3

least 1–1 ½ g per day of cannabis and still having great difficulty in relaxing. She is demanding that she be prescribed the new "ketamine medication I can inhale" because she states, "I need to feel better!" Mrs. X describes her difficulty in sleeping as sleep latency despite her assurance that she practices good sleep hygiene; however, she has difficulty in always remembering to get to bed at the same time, although she states that smoking cannabis nightly was always reliable until lately.

Mrs. X also reports that since she was last into the clinic 3 months ago, her sleep-wake cycles have been so disrupted that she began smoking more cannabis to get to sleep. In doing so, within the past 2 months, paranoia and hallucination began. Also, she reports that since she was last into the clinic 3 months ago, her sleep-wake cycles have been so disrupted that she began smoking more cannabis to get to sleep, and she states that is when, in the past 2 months, the paranoia and hallucinations began. Mrs. X is currently taking oxcarbazepine, and venlafaxine for mood but is also under the care of a pain management specialist who prescribes for her Robaxin, ibuprofen, and gabapentin for her chronic pain syndrome and occasional sumatriptan for migraine headaches. The patient denies having undergone any testing such as computed tomography (CT) scan or magnetic resonance imaging (MRI) of the brain for headaches or memory issues.

Clinical Examination

The patient is a 58-year-old casually dressed Caucasian female with mildly elevated blood pressure (158/85) and BMI 30.6, an increase from 29.4 3-months prior (↑0.8 in 3 months). Physical exam shows no abnormalities of the heart, lungs, and gastrointestinal, dermatological, or musculoskeletal system. The patient admits to intermittent headaches, frequent insomnia with difficulty getting to sleep and staying asleep, increased anxiety, extreme irritability expressed as anger and frustration, feeling down, and feeling "desperate to feel better." She says she feels more forgetful "lately" but denies any history of memory loss or diagnoses associated with neurocognitive disorders. Mrs. X admits to mild hair loss and underlying tiredness. The patient denies active visual hallucinations, auditory hallucinations, and suicidal or homicidal thoughts or behaviors. She has some paranoia as she feels that some people are "out to get me because they know what I have" but abstains from further comments.

Diagnostic Testing

The patient underwent diagnostic testing of routine labs, including basic metabolic panel, HbA$_{1C}$, thyroid function tests, liver function tests, and complete blood counts, in addition to a 10-panel drug screen as a normal part of the patient encounter.

Results of Testing

The patient was found to have a normal complete blood count and basic metabolic panel, except for elevated serum glucose (**150** mg/dL). In addition to the hyperglycemia, the patient laboratory values showed an elevated HbA_{1C} (**7.2%**), cholesterol (**234** mg/dL), high-density lipoprotein cholesterol (HDL-C) (**42** mg/dL), low-density lipoprotein (LDL) (**162** mg/dL), and borderline triglycerides (**178** mmol/L) [1]. Remaining liver function tests were within normal limits.

Also, the patient underwent testing for substance use per routine quarterly visits to ensure compliance with medication prescriptions. According to the US Department of Health and Human Services [2], the patient tested positive for marijuana metabolites (**60** ng/mL, initial test) and a GC-MS confirmatory test for delta-9-tetrahydrocannabinol-9-carboxylic acid ($\triangle^9$-THC) (**17** ng/mL).

Further Investigations

The findings of mild hair loss, tiredness, and increased symptoms of depression, along with an elevated TSH, warrant additional testing to rule out the underlying presence of hypothyroidism superimposed on bipolar depression. While this is likely not a substantial impact on the patient's current condition, it should be corrected to reduce the chances of becoming a problem.

Diagnosis

Based on the clinical history and physical and mental status exams, daily cannabis intake with an increase in recent months, increased anxiety, difficulty sleeping, and sleep deprivation-induced visual hallucinations, a diagnosis of cannabis-induced sleep disorder is confirmed. The benzodiazepine withdrawal may have reasonably precipitated the physiological need to increase cannabis intake resulting in tolerance but also promoting the potential for cannabis intoxication and withdrawal syndrome when the same amount and quality were not consistently ingested. Cannabis use can result in anxiety, irritability, aggression, anger, depressed mood, and difficulty sleeping [3], and given the quality of cannabis currently available on the drug market, monitoring of confiscated cannabis (January 1, 1995, to December 31, 2014) has shown an 8% increase in average THC levels owing to an increase in neurobehavioral features associated with cannabis [4].

Discussion

The effects of cannabis on sleep are variable and dependent on acute versus chronic use of the substance, quality of the substance, route of ingestion, and quantity of the substance. Sedative effects, that are mild in nature, can be noted with the use of low-dose THC along with a decrease in sleep latency [5, 6], at medium to high doses a potential sedative effect [4], and at high-dose ingestion of THC has been found to result in decreased REM, increased sleep latency, slow-wave sleep, and hallucinations [6, 7]. Also, when THC is associated with cannabidiol (CBD), the result is a reduction in slow-wave sleep, a critical issue in learning and memory consolidation [4, 5]. Chronic users of cannabis find little long-term benefits in sleep quality related to resultant anxiety, depression, and overall poor sleep quality [8]. Only acute intoxication with cannabis appears to favor beneficial effects on sleep.

Non-rapid eye movement (NREM) sleep may be intact in this patient, but as she emerges from this phase, hallucinations may present, resulting in anxiety and further awakening, thereby affecting sleepiness, and a pattern of insomnia persists. Aside from anxiety produced by hallucinations, this patient has significantly increased depression from previously, which can result in striking rapid eye movement (REM) sleep disruptions historically noted [9].

Pathophysiology

Cannabinoid (CB) receptors 1 and 2 make up in part the endocannabinoid system (ECS) and include both endogenous and phytocannabinoids, the latter most notably THC [7]. High concentrations of cannabinoid CB1 receptors are found in the basal ganglia, frontal cortex, and cerebellum of the brain. These receptors are responsible for the psychotropic effects of cannabis [6]. Nabiximols, an herbal preparation containing the non-psychoactive cannabinoid extract of THC, cannabidiol (CBD), which is known to interact with G-protein-coupled CB1 receptors in the central nervous system (CNS), results in symptoms of anxiolytic, analgesic effects, and anticonvulsant effects favoring use of these over THC [4, 10].

Sleep Disturbance

Long-term use of cannabis for medicinal therapy, recreational therapy, or both can result in dependence in one of two daily users. In a trial of drug withdrawal, cannabis users experienced intense sleep disturbances noted as nightmares or strange dreams, angry outbursts during sleep, early awakening, and trouble getting to sleep, the latter a common finding in most substance withdrawal studies [7, 11, 12]. The use of synthetic cannabis (SC) shows a similar pattern and may, therefore, further promote increasing use to stem anxiety, visual hallucinations, and sleep deprivation [4].

Several studies of polysomnography (PSG) in short periods of cannabis use report shorter sleep latency (SL), decreased time awake after sleep onset (WASO), increased slow-wave sleep (SWS), and decreased rapid eye movement REM. In chronic users of cannabis, they develop tolerance to most effects observed in short-term use, including its sleep-inducing effects and slow-wave sleep enhancement.

Sleep efficiency is similarly unimproved or worsens. PSG studies of cannabis withdrawal have demonstrated an increase in sleep onset latency and wakefulness after sleep onset. Total sleep time, sleep efficiency, and slow-wave sleep time are reduced, and REM sleep is increased (REM rebound). Shorter REM latency has also been reported [13].

Insomnia

The ability to fully understand the impact of THC and CBD on sleep quality in humans has primarily been based on self-reports and thus conflicting at times. Hence, an increase in prevalence rate may not be exact; however, it is safe to say that there has been an increase in the prevalence rate of insomnia (19.2%), defined as difficulty in falling asleep and/or maintaining sleep, and/or dissatisfaction with the quality of sleep such that there is significant distress or impairment in functioning [7]. Correlates between those using cannabis for medical purposes (pain) indicate that most (80%) used cannabis to help with sleep, which more frequently resulted in cannabis withdrawal symptoms [14].

Sleep difficulties appear to be a predisposing factor for cannabis use, and baseline sleep problem is a significant predictor of later cannabis use, doubling the risk of future use. Higher rates of relapse have been correlated with poor sleep quality and other withdrawal symptoms [12].

Chronic Pain

Approximately 20% of adults struggle with chronic pain affecting their ability to obtain adequate quality sleep. Recent literature suggests the use of a 1:1 THC/CBD preparation did not support an increase in sleep duration as opposed to a synthetic THC preparation. Additional research is needed to determine if synthetic preparations of THC alone, as opposed to amitriptyline, result in improved sleep among fibromyalgia patients who traditionally suffer from poor sleep quality [7].

Pearls
1. Chronic cannabis users can increase the likelihood of developing anxiety, depression, and significant sleep disturbance with increasing intake problems.
2. Consider cannabis withdrawal syndrome for symptoms of extreme irritability/anger, anxiety, depression, and sleep disturbances.
3. Cannabis intake has a variable impact on the quality of sleep and is dependent on several factors, including whether the person is cannabis naive, the quality of cannabis, the quantity of cannabis, and the method of intake.

References

1. Fischbach FT, Fischbach MA. Fischbach's: a manual of laboratory and diagnostic tests. 10th ed. Baltimore: Wolters Kluwer; 2018.
2. U. S. Department of Health and Human Services. Mandatory guidelines for federal workplace drug testing programs. Federal Register. 2017;82(13). http://www.samhsa.gov/workplace/drugtesting.
3. American Psychiatric Association. Diagnostic and statistical manual of mental disorders. 5th ed. Washington, DC: American Psychiatric Association; 2013.
4. Lafaye G, Karila L, Blecha L, Benyamina A. Pharmacological aspects: cannabis, cannabinoids, and health. Dialogues Clin Neurosci. 2017;19(3):309–16.
5. Garcia AN, Salloum IM. Polysomnographic sleep disturbances in nicotine, caffeine, alcohol, cocaine, opioid, and cannabis use: a focused review. Am J Addict. 2015;24(7):590–8. https://doi.org/10.1111/ajad.12291.
6. National Academies of Sciences, Engineering, and Medicine. The health effects of cannabis and cannabinoids: the current state of evidence and recommendations for research. National Academies. 2017. https://doi.org/10.17226/24625.
7. Babson K, Sottile J, Morabito D. Cannabis, cannabinoids, and sleep: a review of the literature. Curr Psychiatry Rep. 2017;19(23):1–12. https://doi.org/10.1007/s11920-017-0775-9.
8. Hser Y, Mooney LJ, Huang D, Zhu Y, Tomko RL, McClure E, et al. Reductions in cannabis use are associated with improvements in anxiety, depression, and sleep quality, but not the quality of life. J Subst Abus Treat. 2017;81:53–8. https://doi.org/10.1016/j.jsat.2017.07.012.
9. Sadock B, Sadock V, Ruiz P. Kaplan & Sadock's concise textbook of clinical psychiatry. 4th ed. Philadelphia: Wolters Kluwer; 2017.
10. PubChem. (n.d.). Compound summary: nabiximols. *U.S. National Library of Medicine, National Center for Biotechnology Information.* Retrieved from https://pubchem.ncbi.nlm.nih.gov/compound/Nabiximols.
11. Allsop DJ, Norberg MM, Copeland J, Fu S, Budney AJ. The Cannabis Withdrawal scale development: patterns and predictors of cannabis withdrawal and distress. Drug Alcohol Depend. 2011;119:123–9. https://doi.org/10.1016/j.drugalcdep.2011.06.003.
12. Schierenbeck T, Riemann D, Hornyak M, et al. Effects of illicit recreational drugs upon sleep: cocaine, ecstasy, and marijuana. Sleep Med Rev. 2008;12(5):381–9.
13. Vandrey R, Smith MT, al CEM e. Sleep disturbances and the effects of extended-release zolpidem during Cannabis withdrawal. Drug Alcohol Depend. 2011;117(1):38–44.
14. Cranford JA, Arnedt JT, Conroy DA, Bohnert KM, Bourque C, Blow FC, Ilgen M. Prevalence and correlates of sleep-related problems in adults receiving medical cannabis for chronic pain. Drug Alcohol Depend. 2017;180:227–33. https://doi.org/10.1016/j.drugalcdep.2017.08.017.

People Think Alcohol Helps with Sleep

4

Joseph Westermeyer, Patricia Dickmann, and Heather Swanson

Clinical History/Case

A 71-year-old married retired man presented with the complaint, "My sleep isn't good." He had difficulty falling asleep and staying asleep over the previous 3–4 months. His primary care physician had prescribed diphenhydramine 50 mg several years ago with good effect, but it was not helping him at this time. A course of trazodone 100 mg likewise failed to relieve his insomnia. Consequently, he had begun drinking one bottle of beer every night to aid falling asleep. His eldest brother, aged 83, had died recently. Providing daycare for two grandchildren, ages 3 and 5, "tired him out" by the end of the day over the last several months, resulting in daytime fatigue. His wife had recently been diagnosed as having obstructive sleep apnea (OSA); she was receiving nighttime continuous positive airway pressure (CPAP) with excellent results. She reported that he snored heavily "for many years" and had breathing cessations.

Past Medical History His current health conditions included hypertension and gastroesophageal reflux. Three months previously a medication regimen for hepatitis C (sofosbuvir-ribavirin) had rendered him antigen negative. He was a chronic tobacco smoker who complained of episodic low back pain. Past mental health problems included alcohol use disorder (AUD) during early adulthood, with several later

J. Westermeyer (✉) · P. Dickmann · H. Swanson
Department of Psychiatry, University of Minnesota, Minneapolis VA Health Care Center, Minneapolis, MN, USA

Mental Health, Minneapolis VA Medical Center, Minneapolis, MN, USA

Addiction Recovery Services, Minneapolis Veterans Affairs Medical Center, Minneapolis, MN, USA
e-mail: joseph.westermeyer@va.gov

© Springer Nature Switzerland AG 2021
I. S. Khawaja, T. D. Hurwitz (eds.), *Sleep Disorders in Selected Psychiatric Settings*, https://doi.org/10.1007/978-3-030-59309-4_4

recurrences that responded to treatment. His last AUD relapse occurred at age 69, when he developed acute pancreatitis while on vacation. He developed combat-related posttraumatic stress disorder, including nightmares involving the combat death of a close friend in Vietnam. Psychotherapy and prazosin relieved his post-traumatic symptoms in recent years. During middle age, he had developed major depressive disorder (MDD), which responded to fluoxetine 40 mg. When his MDD failed to respond to selective serotonin reuptake inhibitor (SSRI)s in his mid-60s, he ultimately responded to augmentation therapy of fluoxetine with aripiprazole 15 mg daily.

Medications This patient was prescribed lisinopril, amlodipine, and omeprazole for his hypertension and reflux. After experiencing excellent relief of his chronic posttraumatic stress disorder (PTSD) and depressive symptoms with the aid of pra-zosin, fluoxetine, and aripiprazole, he allowed these prescriptions to lapse. He sub-sequently experienced recent return of psychiatric symptoms (i.e., anxiety, suspiciousness, mistrust, dreams related to two tours in Vietnam with the Marines).

Family History There was no family history of substance use or mental health issues. In addition, there was no family history of obstructive sleep apnea (OSA), narcolepsy, restless legs syndrome (RLS), or other sleep disorders.

Review of Systems On initial evaluation, he reported the following symptoms: ini-tial and middle insomnia, excessive daytime sleepiness with frequent dozing, and observed snoring and "snort arousals" per his wife. He denied symptoms consistent with cataplexy, hypnagogic or hypnopompic hallucinations, or sleep paralysis.

Social History He lived in a small Midwestern town with his wife in their own home. They owned a condominium in Florida, where they vacationed with their children and grandchildren. A college graduate, he had worked at various occupa-tions during his life. During the worst of his post-trauma symptoms, drinking, and depression following Vietnam, he and his wife had been separated for years. He described himself currently as a "hands-on grandfather" who was actively involved with his extended family. In association with his own multiethnic background (Native American, Scots-Irish, and African American) and his personal military experience, he was interested in the histories of ethnic units in the US military.

Examination/Mental Status Exam

His BMI was 33.1 (height, 71 inches; weight, 237 pounds). He had no other perti-nent physical findings.

Differential Diagnoses
- Obstructive sleep apnea (OSA) [1]
- Central sleep apnea (CSA) [1]

- Hypoxemia secondary to chronic tobacco use [4]
- PTSD or MDD-related insomnia. [8, 9]

Special Studies Gamma glutyamyl transpeptidase (GGT), serum glutamyl oxalocetic transaminase (SGOT), serum glytamyl pyruvate transaminase (SGPT), creatinine, complete blood cell count, urinalysis, urine drug screen, overnight sleep electroencephalographic (EEG) study, and sleep questionnaires [2–6].

Results Since treatment for hepatitis C, his GGT had normalized; SGOT and SGPT were improving. Creatinine was slightly elevated and stable at 1.4 mg%. Complete blood count, routine urinalysis, and urine drug screen were normal. Watch-PAT was notable for the following values: 102.2 PAT Respiratory Disturbance Index (PRDI) and 66.0 Oxygen Desaturation Index (ODI). $SpO_2\%$ was a mean of 96% (89% minimum). PAT Valid Sleep Time (PVST) was 8 hours 54 minutes.

Final Sleep Clinic Diagnosis Severe obstructive sleep apnea. It was recommended that he start auto-titrating positive airway pressure (APAP) [7].

Follow-Up Our first intervention focused on his alcohol use, since his previous AUD had caused social alienation from his wife and extended family, as well as producing life-threatening pancreatitis. The patient was willing to re-establish sobriety and take naltrexone for the evolving alcohol cravings. He returned to clinic weekly while gradually titrating naltrexone to 150 mg daily. His ethnic imperatives (Scots-Irish and Native American cultures) urged him to drink in the evening with his daughter, since drinking alone was considered risky and could be antisocial. Around this time, her new job enabled her to move to an apartment nearby. This enabled the patient to care for his grandchildren, while avoiding a bedtime libation with his daughter. He had agreed to an intensive outpatient program if he could not sustain abstinence, but this alternative proved unnecessary.

He was willing to resume prazosin for Vietnam-related dreams. Resumption of fluoxetine and aripiprazole augmentation relieved his suspiciousness and reduced, but did not eliminate, his nighttime awakening and daytime fatigue. Weekly mindfulness training over 3 months helped him in coping with the recent loss of his elder brother, as well as the death of his friend in combat decades ago. Mindfulness training empowered him as an actor in his own recovery (rather than relying solely on interventions impressed by clinicians).

Following confirmation of OSA diagnosis, initiation of APAP eliminated his nighttime insomnia and gradually alleviated his daytime fatigue (along with fluoxetine and aripiprazole). His wife reported that APAP alleviated his snoring. He continued providing daycare for his grandchildren – an important factor in bolstering his self-esteem, confidence, and the meaningfulness of his life. Although initially he doubted that he and his wife could have the same sleep malady, his familiarity with her treatment, course, and improvement aided his understanding of the disorder and his compliance with treatment.

Question What caused this patient's initial insomnia, nighttime awakenings, and daytime fatigue?

Discussion Several factors could account for his recent initial insomnia, awakening during the night, and daytime fatigue. Caring for his active grandsons at age 71 began around the same time as his daytime fatigue. He may have accommodated to his bedtime dose of antihistaminic diphenhydramine for initial insomnia. Following 2 years of abstinence following life-threatening pancreatitis, he had resumed mild alcohol use for bedtime sedation. Even mild alcohol use, taken regularly, could produce rapid eye movement (REM) abnormalities in an older man. PTSD-related dreams had recently resumed, in association with his decision to discontinue prazosin for nightmares. He had likewise discontinued aripiprazole on his own – an augmentation regimen that had relieved his treatment-refractory MDD. In addition, his eldest brother had recently died – a close friend and the first of his siblings to die. A prolonged grief reaction could have precipitated a mood disorder. His initial insomnia could possibly ensue from relapse to his anxiety disorder (PTSD), and later reawakening every hour or two could result from recurrence of his mood disorder (MDD).

Failure to address these coexisting problems early on could complicate additional sleep evaluation as well as sleep-related interventions. Since it would require several weeks before a sleep consultation with sleep laboratory assessment could be accomplished, we had sufficient time to address his coexisting problems. From his own past clinical experiences, and his recent observations of his wife's CPAP treatment for OSA, he understood the clinical challenges lying ahead. Despite his original doubts that he could have OSA like his wife, his familiarity with her sleep assessment and treatment was helpful in preparing him for his own evaluation and care for a sleep disorder. Thus, we were able to mobilize his willingness to address the diverse conditions that might complicate his sleep diagnoses and undermine future sleep interventions.

Pearls
- Sleep disorders can be multifactorial in etiology, i.e., substance use, anxiety disorder, mood disorder, and bereavement.
- The phased nature of his SUD-PTSD-MDD-bereavement treatment helped in preparation for sleep consultation, diagnostic evaluation, and CPAP treatment.
- It is important to have awareness of the generational and sociocultural attitudes and values of this patient. In this case, the importance of (1) his relationships with his daughter, her children, his wife, and his extended family as being central to his care and (2) his need for active involvement in his own treatment and recovery plan, so as to sustain his self-esteem and enhance his personal power.

References

1. American Academy of Sleep Medicine. International classification of sleep disorders. 3rd ed. Darian: American Academy of Sleep Medicine; 2014.
2. Buysse DJ, Reynolds CF, Monk TH, Berman SR, Kupfer DJ. The Pittsburgh sleep quality index: a new instrument for psychiatric practice and research. Psychiatry Res. 1989;28:193–213.
3. Colraine IM, Turlington S, Baker FC. Impact of alcoholism on sleep architecture and EEG power spectra in men and women. Sleep. 2009;32(10):1341–52.
4. Currie SR, Clark S, Rimac S, Malhotra S. Comprehensive assessment of insomnia in recovery alcoholics using daily sleep diaries and ambulatory monitoring. Alcohol Clin Exp Res. 2003;27(8):1262–9.
5. Farney RJ, McDonald AM, Boyle KM, Snow GL, Nuttall RT, Coudreaut MF, et al. Sleep disordered breathing in patients receiving therapy. Eur Respir J. 2013;42:394–403.
6. Johns MW. A new method of measuring daytime sleepiness: the Epworth Sleepiness Scale. Sleep. 1991;14:540–5.
7. Stein MD, Friedmann PD. Disturbed sleep and its relationship to alcohol use. Subst Abus. 2005;26:1): 1–13.
8. Westermeyer JJ, Khawaja IS, et al. Correlates of daytime sleepiness in patients with posttraumatic stress disorder and sleep disturbance. Prim Care Companion J Clin Psychiatry. 2010;12:2.
9. Westermeyer JJ, Khawaja IS, et al. Quality of sleep in patients with posttraumatic stress disorder. Psychiatry. 2010;7(9):21–7.

When Counting Sheep Doesn't Help: The Effects of Cocaine on Sleep

Nidal Moukaddam and Asim A. Shah

History

Ms. D. is a 28-year-old female who presents to clinic asking for help with anxiety and insomnia at night. She reports that she used drugs from ages 18 to 27 and has recently become abstinent after a course of inpatient rehabilitation. She has been working full-time and is very happy to be a productive member of society again. She works from 9 am to 5 pm most days but has late shifts until 10 pm once or twice per week. On those days, she finds it even harder to fall asleep.

The patient denies any acute or chronic medical illnesses. She denies a history of trauma and nightmares; she had a brief episode of depression as a teenager but has not been depressed since becoming sober. She has no anhedonia and had no neuro-vegetative symptoms except poor sleep. Her appetite was slightly increased. She felt sleepy and tired often during the day. She never has psychotic symptoms and never developed hopelessness or suicidal ideations.

Ms. D describes a period after she stopped using drugs during which her sleep improved. However, her partner noted that she was kicking a lot during the night and seemed to not be resting comfortably. This stage lasted ~2 weeks followed by worsening of her feelings of insomnia.

N. Moukaddam (✉)
Department of Psychiatry and Behavioral Sciences, Baylor College of Medicine, Houston, TX, USA
e-mail: nidalm@bcm.edu

A. A. Shah
Menninger Department of Psychiatry and Behavioral Sciences, Baylor College of Medicine, Houston, TX, USA

© Springer Nature Switzerland AG 2021
I. S. Khawaja, T. D. Hurwitz (eds.), *Sleep Disorders in Selected Psychiatric Settings*, https://doi.org/10.1007/978-3-030-59309-4_5

Exam/Mental Status

- *Vital signs: HR 110, BP 110/80, RR 16, O$_2$ saturation 100% on RA*
- Patient has a normal body mass index (BMI)
- *Constitutional:* No acute distress. Person, place, situation and date × 3
- *HEENT:* PERRL, EOMI, no nasal discharge, pharynx non-erythematous
- *Neck:* Trachea midline, FROM no JVD. No cervical lymphadenopathy
- *Cardiac:* Heart regular rhythm without murmurs, rubs, or gallops
- *Respiratory:* Lungs clear to auscultation bilaterally. No accessory muscles used in breathing. No tachypnea. No wheezes or rhonchi or rales
- *Abdomen:* Soft, non-tender. Non-distended. No organomegaly. Normoactive bowel sounds
- *Musculoskeletal:* No joint effusions or erythema. Grossly full active range of motion. No distal edema in lower extremities. Dorsalis pedis and posterior tibial pulses 2+ bilaterally
- *Neuro:* Cranial nerves II–XII grossly intact. Strength 5/5 bilaterally in upper and lower extremities. Sensation grossly intact to light touch bilaterally in upper and lower extremities
- *Skin:* No rashes. No jaundice

Mental Status Exam

The patient presents as a thin but well-nourished adult female in casual clothes. She makes good eye contact with the examiner and is appropriately cooperative. She has tattoos of butterflies on her neck, but lesions, track marks, or other markings.

Affect was appropriate to interview, with mild anxiety. The patient described her mood as "good." Thought process was linear, coherent, and goal directed, and thought content was negative for psychosis, suicidality, or intent to harm others. Her memory, attention span, abstraction level, and fund of knowledge were within normal limits.

Tests

This patient was seen for an initial assessment and two follow-up visits. Polysomnography (PSG), sleep diary, and blood work were ordered.

Results

Blood work obtained at initial visit included a complete blood count, electrolytes, thyroid panel, and renal and liver function tests, which were all within normal.

The patient was asked to fill a sleep diary for 2 weeks. Findings reveal interrupted sleep, with total hours of sleep between 4 and 6 hours per night and two to four awakenings per night, sometimes related to bad dreams. The patient specified when asked the dreams were not related to past events (no re-enactment).

Polysomnography

Comprehensive polysomnography was performed. This included recording electro-encephalogram, electro-oculograms, submentalis electromyogram, anterior tibialis movement sensor, and electrocardiogram.

The total recording period was 367.5 minutes. The total sleep time was 313.0 minutes with a sleep efficiency of 85.2%. Sleep onset latency was 0.0 minutes. Latency to persistent sleep (10 minutes of uninterrupted sleep) was 4.0 minutes. Arousals and awakenings occurred on an average of 9.8 per hour, and sleep architecture was fragmented. The patient had 0.0% delta sleep. Rapid eye movement (REM) latency was 62 minutes, and REM sleep was 15.0% of total sleep time. The total time awake after sleep onset was 54.5 minutes.

EEG Characteristics: During wakefulness, the dominant occipital rhythm was 8–13 Hz and was symmetric and reactive to eye opening. Expected REM and non-REM characteristics were recorded.

This patient's report highlighted several abnormalities including:

- Sleep continuity deterioration and fragmentation
- Decrease in total sleep time
- Decrease in sleep efficiency
- Increase in sleep onset time
- Decrease in REM duration
- Slow wave sleep decrease that was not age-appropriate

Question *What is the effect of cocaine on sleep? Is there a preferred treatment? Should I treat or reassure the patient the insomnia is time limited?*

Differential Diagnosis
In this case, the clinician is invited to consider primary insomnia, cocaine-induced sleep disorder, insomnia type, and primary sleep disorders, e.g., primary insomnia, being unmasked by current cocaine abstinence. Illicit use of other stimulants also figures on the differential diagnosis list.

Discussion In the following sections, we will look at the effects of cocaine on sleep and the diagnostic considerations the clinician must keep in mind.

Cocaine History and Demographics

Cocaine (benzoylmethylecgonine) is derived from coca leaves, a plant indigenous to the Andes Mountains. Coca leaves have been used for centuries as a stimulant and a mild to moderate appetite suppressant: in that context, the leaves are chewed or made into tea. Cocaine extracts were added into drinks around the turn of the twentieth century. Half-life is 4–7 hours, depending on repeated administration [1]. Illicit use cocaine has chnaged: until late 1970s, early 1980s, use was predominantly related to cocaine (hydrochloride) powder insufflation or injection; in the 1980s, the crack cocaine epidemic (cocaine alkaloids) became a significant public health issue [2, 3].

Cocaine is a psychoactive drug with psychomimetic effects. Cocaine effects are complex and not limited to one neurotransmitter system; main action is mediated via action on monoamines (inverse agonism of the dopamine transporter) [4, 5] leading to depletion in dopamine, but glutamatergic action has been more of a focus in recent years [6] as well as its effects on hippocampal neurogenesis [7].

Clinical Manifestations Use leads to a high characterized [8] by euphoria, activation, and at least two of the following: tachycardia or bradycardia, pupillary dilation, fluctuations in blood pressure, sweating or chills, nausea/vomiting, suppressed appetite (with weight loss in the context of repeated use), and psychomotor changes; use may also lead to muscular weakness, respiratory depression, chest pain, or cardiac arrhythmias, confusion, seizures, or coma.

Cocaine use is sustained, despite the popularity of other drugs (opioids, amphetamines) that have eclipsed it slightly in the past few years. Studies on global burden of disease attributable to cocaine show that countries with highest incomes have the highest rates of burden, with steeper use in adolescence and early adulthood [9]. The National Survey on Drug Use and Health (NSDUH) estimates past year cocaine use in young adults to be close to 5%, with wide variations across states [10].

Users often use adulterated cocaine without their knowledge, and the top adulterants were found to be levamisole, phenacetin, lidocaine, hydroxyzine, and diltiazem [11]. It remains the highest reason for drug-related emergency room visits because it can cause hypertension, myocardial ischemia and infarction, and acute aortic dissection.

Among substance users, sleep disturbances including insomnia, hypersomnia, or both are reported by almost half of individuals surveyed [12], and the severity of sleep disturbance correlated with more severe substance use at entry into treatment programs. Sleep disturbance was still reported after 12 months of drug abstinence [12].

How to Diagnose a Stimulant-Induced Sleep Disorder?

In the ICD-10 and the DSM-5, cocaine is classified under the category of stimulants as they share common pharmacological profile and clinical actions. According to the DSM-5, a stimulant-induced sleep disorder is diagnosed when "a prominent and severe disturbance in sleep" occurs during or soon after substance intoxication or after withdrawal from or exposure to the substance, as indicated by history, physical exam, or laboratory findings [8]. Subtypes and specifiers for the cocaine-induced sleep disorder include insomnia type, daytime sleepiness type, parasomnia type, and mixed type. Care must also be taken to include the diagnosis of a substance use disorder when applicable. In most cases, substance use that is severe enough to cause a sleep disorder often meets the criteria for a full substance use disorder (misuse/abuse/dependence). In diagnosing a stimulant-induced disorder, delirium, other medical issues, and other sleep disorders preceding the substance use must be excluded. The duration of stimulant-induced sleep disorder is at least a month.

General Cocaine-Related Sleep Effects

Dopamine, serotonin, and norepinephrine are involved in sleep regulation, with dopamine being the only active neurotransmitter during REM sleep. Dopaminergic tone is involved in wakefulness, and a reduction in dopaminergic tone leads to drowsiness, enhancing sleep [13]. Chronic use of stimulants including cocaine lowers monoaminergic tones, and abstinence leads to rebound REM and decreased REM latency. However, increased dopamine (rebound) also may lead to vivid, nightmarish dreams. Although direct evidence is lacking, insomnia (and often accompanying anxiety at night) is thought to increase chances [14, 15] of relapse in drug users. Outcomes of individual users may depend on depressive symptoms as well as sleep disturbances in exploratory studies [16].

Very few studies have employed polysomnography to document sleep dysregulation, though those symptoms are commonly noted in clinical practice. As reviewed by Valladares [17], sleep abnormalities akin to those listed in the polysomnography section above are very common.

Cognitive effects following abstinence from cocaine and associated sleep issues include difficulties with attention and sleep-dependent learning [18]. In a study by Trksak et al., correlating magnetic resonance spectroscopy (MRS) brain imaging, polysomnography, and Continuous Performance Task with Digit Symbol Substitution Task, cocaine-dependent individuals performed more poorly on the cognitive tasks listed above, even in the absence of sleep deprivation [19].

Translated into clinical perspective, this may be reported by the patient as difficulty focusing on their often newly acquired employment or daytime occupations and increase of risk of loss of these positions, further exacerbating risk for relapse.

Sleep Disturbances During Active Drug Use

During the active phase of use of cocaine, activation is accompanied by absence of sleep or diminished sleep [20], and this ability to stay awake and alert constitutes one of the attractive features of cocaine use for individuals choosing it. During that time, sleep architecture is disturbed as follows: the total amount of sleep is reduced, sleep latency is increased as patients stay up even after the euphoria starts to fade and cannot fall asleep, and sleep continuity is disrupted, and the total amount of REM sleep is decreased.

The 24 hours or so following cocaine intoxication are characterized by hypersomnia and increased appetite, and these effects can persist for up to a week, depending on how physiologically dependent the user is. Repeated cocaine use will exacerbate the insomnia and may contribute to the development of paranoia. Sleep specialists rarely see cocaine users during the acute phase of sleep disturbances.

Hypersomnia during early abstinence co-occurs with dysphoria, and evidence suggests that hypersomnia worsens cravings [15].

Cocaine-Related Sleep Disturbances During the Abstinence Phase

Following the first few days of abstinence from cocaine, most users report a subjective improvement in sleep that is not reflected in polysomnographic measures or in cognitive tests [21]. This phenomenon is termed *occult insomnia*. Occult insomnia may lead to relapse, and clinicians need to be aware that brief subjective progress in sleep is not indicative of normalization of sleep architecture [21]; thus, patients will still be at risk of relapse and other issues arising from cocaine sequelae even in the absence of active drug consumption. The period between the first week and third week of abstinence may carry the best subjective sleep reports.

Rebound in REM sleep, associated with bad dreams, may be a treatment target in the early weeks of abstinence [21]. Cocaine users also display loss of Stage 3 sleep compared to age-matched controls [22].

Potential Treatments in Cocaine-Induced Insomnia

In the context of cocaine-induced insomnia, psychotropic agents that have sedating properties may be desirable, and they help with both sleep and cocaine cravings. In an animal experiment by Chen et al., manipulation of sleep architecture was effective in reducing cocaine relapses in study subjects even when total sleep time was left unchanged (and below normal levels) [15]. This area is relatively understudied, as both improvements in REM and non-REM sleep are associated with general improvement; it is unclear to what extent the decrease in sleep fragmentation or the improvement in stress due to sleep deprivation contributes to decrease in cocaine-seeking behaviors. The molecular targets of cocaine-induced insomnia and general dysfunction are also wide-ranging: as mentioned above, monoamines participate in sleep regulation; the glutamatergic system is also a contributor. Additionally, the orexin/hypocretin system is a viable target for treatments: orexins regulate stimulation and reward. Mechanistic considerations dictate improvement, but increasing total sleep time, e.g., via GABAergic agents, is not enough: in a small study by Morgan et al., comparing tiagabine and lorazepam suggests that lorazepam, despite increasing total sleep time, entailed worsening in cognitive effects and impulsivity the day post-administration, whereas tiagabine increased slow wave sleep [23].

Dual orexin receptor antagonists (DORAs) such as suvorexant, approved for treatment of insomnia, have shown promise in mitigating cocaine cravings and cocaine-seeking behaviors in animals [24]. Human studies are currently underway.

Mirtazapine, with antagonism at the $5-HT_{2A}$ receptor, was found to be helpful in depressive disorders occurring concomitantly with cocaine use disorder [25] but did not help with decreasing cocaine use. Quetiapine, a second-generation antipsychotic, was found to help with anxiety and sleep in substance use disorders (cocaine as well as other drugs), an improvement thought to be mediated by sleep normalization [26].

Modafinil, which shares some cocaine actions in terms of dopamine transporter blockade and has both stimulant and appetite suppression effects, promotes wakefulness and regulates circadian rhythms, helps with daytime drowsiness, and also has evidence in decreasing relapse on cocaine [27]. Modafinil normalizes sleep parameters in previous cocaine users [28].

Pearls
- Cocaine use is common and sleep disturbances occur during active use and after drug abstinence.
- Cocaine abstinence is associated with sleep issues that impair cognition, memory, attention, and procedural learning.
- Cocaine-associated sleep disturbances include change in total sleep duration, REM sleep, sleep efficiency, and slow wave decrease.
- Poor sleep outcomes may be associated with higher odds of relapse.
- No approved treatment for cocaine-induced insomnia exists though modafinil, a cognitive enhancer thought to work through dopamine receptor blockade, shows promise in sleep architecture normalization and improvement in sustained abstinence.

References

1. Inaba T, Stewart DJ, Kalow W. Metabolism of cocaine in man. Clin Pharmacol Ther. 1978;23(5):547–52.
2. Parker MA, Anthony JC. Should anyone be riding to glory on the now-descending limb of the crack-cocaine epidemic curve in the United States? Drug Alcohol Depend. 2014;138:225–8.

3. Tsuchiya H. Anesthetic agents of plant origin: a review of phytochemicals with anesthetic activity. Molecules (Basel, Switzerland). 2017;22(8).
4. Heal DJ, Gosden J, Smith SL. Dopamine reuptake transporter (DAT) "inverse agonism" – a novel hypothesis to explain the enigmatic pharmacology of cocaine. Neuropharmacology. 2014;87:19–40.
5. Schmitt KC, Rothman RB, Reith ME. Nonclassical pharmacology of the dopamine transporter: atypical inhibitors, allosteric modulators, and partial substrates. J Pharmacol Exp Ther. 2013;346(1):2–10.
6. Marquez J, Campos-Sandoval JA, Penalver A, et al. Glutamate and brain glutaminases in drug addiction. Neurochem Res. 2017;42(3):846–57.
7. Castilla-Ortega E, Ladron de Guevara-Miranda D, Serrano A, et al. The impact of cocaine on adult hippocampal neurogenesis: potential neurobiological mechanisms and contributions to maladaptive cognition in cocaine addiction disorder. Biochem Pharmacol. 2017;141:100–17.
8. Substance-Related and Addictive Disorders. *Diagnostic and statistical manual of mental disorders.*
9. Degenhardt L, Whiteford HA, Ferrari AJ, et al. Global burden of disease attributable to illicit drug use and dependence: findings from the Global Burden of Disease Study 2010. Lancet (London, England). 2013;382(9904):1564–74.
10. Hughes A, Williams MR, Lipari RN, Van Horn S. State estimates of past year cocaine use among young adults: 2014 and 2015. *The CBHSQ Report.* Rockville: Substance Abuse and Mental Health Services Administration (US); 2013. p. 1–9.
11. Solimini R, Rotolo MC, Pellegrini M, et al. Adulteration practices of psychoactive illicit drugs: an updated review. Curr Pharm Biotechnol. 2017;18(7):524–30.
12. Dolsen MR, Harvey AG. Life-time history of insomnia and hypersomnia symptoms as correlates of alcohol, cocaine and heroin use and relapse among adults seeking substance use treatment in the United States from 1991 to 1994. Addiction (Abingdon, England). 2017;112(6):1104–11.
13. Agargun MY, Ozbek H. Drug effects on dreaming. In: Sleep and sleep disorders: a neuropsychopharmacological approach. Boston: Springer US; 2006. p. 256–61.
14. Pace-Schott EF, Stickgold R, Muzur A, et al. Sleep quality deteriorates over a binge--abstinence cycle in chronic smoked cocaine users. Psychopharmacology. 2005;179(4):873–83.
15. Chen B, Wang Y, Liu X, Liu Z, Dong Y, Huang YH. Sleep regulates incubation of cocaine craving. J Neurosci Off J Soc Neurosci. 2015;35(39):13300–10.
16. Sofuoglu M, Dudish-Poulsen S, Poling J, Mooney M, Hatsukami DK. The effect of individual cocaine withdrawal symptoms on outcomes in cocaine users. Addict Behav. 2005;30(6):1125–34.
17. Valladares EM, Irwin MR. Polysomnographic sleep dysregulation in cocaine dependence. TheScientificWorldJOURNAL. 2007;7:213–6.
18. Angarita GA, Canavan SV, Forselius E, Bessette A, Pittman B, Morgan PT. Abstinence-related changes in sleep during treatment for cocaine dependence. Drug Alcohol Depend. 2014;134:343–7.
19. Trksak GH, Bracken BK, Jensen JE, et al. Effects of sleep deprivation on brain bioenergetics, sleep, and cognitive performance in cocaine-dependent individuals. TheScientificWorldJOURNAL. 2013;2013:947879.
20. Schierenbeck T, Riemann D, Berger M, Hornyak M. Effect of illicit recreational drugs upon sleep: cocaine, ecstasy and marijuana. Sleep Med Rev. 2008;12(5):381–9.
21. Angarita GA, Emadi N, Hodges S, Morgan PT. Sleep abnormalities associated with alcohol, cannabis, cocaine, and opiate use: a comprehensive review. Addict Sci Clin Pract. 2016;11(1):9.
22. Irwin MR, Bjurstrom MF, Olmstead R. Polysomnographic measures of sleep in cocaine dependence and alcohol dependence: implications for age-related loss of slow wave, stage 3 sleep. Addiction (Abingdon, England). 2016;111(6):1084–92.
23. Morgan PT, Malison RT. Pilot study of lorazepam and tiagabine effects on sleep, motor learning, and impulsivity in cocaine abstinence. Am J Drug Alcohol Abuse. 2008;34(6):692–702.

24. Gentile TA, Simmons SJ, Barker DJ, Shaw JK, Espana RA, Muschamp JW. Suvorexant, an orexin/hypocretin receptor antagonist, attenuates motivational and hedonic properties of cocaine. Addict Biol. 2018;23(1):247–55.
25. Afshar M, Knapp CM, Sarid-Segal O, et al. The efficacy of mirtazapine in the treatment of cocaine dependence with comorbid depression. Am J Drug Alcohol Abuse. 2012;38(2):181–6.
26. Sattar SP, Bhatia SC, Petty F. Potential benefits of quetiapine in the treatment of substance dependence disorders. J Psychiatry Neurosci. 2004;29(6):452–7.
27. Kumar R. Approved and investigational uses of modafinil: an evidence-based review. Drugs. 2008;68(13):1803–39.
28. Morgan PT, Pace-Schott E, Pittman B, Stickgold R, Malison RT. Normalizing effects of modafinil on sleep in chronic cocaine users. Am J Psychiatry. 2010;167(3):331–40.

Part III

Sleep Issues in Pregnancy

Insomnia in Pregnancy

6

Safia S. Khan and Gregory S. Carter

Clinical History

Ms. A. M. was a 36-year-old G1P0 healthy lady at 28 weeks' gestation, who presented to the sleep clinic with difficulty falling asleep and staying asleep since beginning her second trimester. She found herself staying up until 1:00 AM working on her computer or reading journals three to four times a week. She then had difficulty awaking in the morning and excessive daytime fatigue. She tried to go to bed earlier to allow herself more opportunity to sleep; however, she was frustrated by continuing to struggle to initiate sleep. Once asleep, she would wake up three to four times per night due to both acid reflux and a need to check and ascertain if her doors were locked. Her husband reported that for the last 2 months, she occasionally snored at night. Her typical day started at 8:00 AM when she arose with her alarm in order to get to work by 9:00 AM. She had one cup of coffee in the morning and occasionally a soda at dinner. They watched TV after dinner, and then she worked on her computer for an hour or two.

She had a history of difficulty sleeping prior to her exams and midterms but has always excelled in her studies. This previous difficulty sleeping resolved without any medications and only lasted about 4–5 years while she was in college.

S. S. Khan (✉)
Department of Family and Community Medicine, Department of Neurology and Neurotherapeutics at University of Texas Southwestern Medical Center, Dallas, TX, USA

Parkland Sleep Center, Parkland Medical Hospital, Dallas, TX, USA

Texas Health Resources Presbyterian Hospital, Dallas, TX, USA
e-mail: Safia.khan@utsouthwestern.edu

G. S. Carter
UT Southwestern Sleep Medicine Fellowship Program, Department of Neurology and Neurotherapeutics at The University of Texas Southwestern Medical Center at Dallas, Dallas, TX, USA
e-mail: Gregory.carter@utsouthwestern.edu

© Springer Nature Switzerland AG 2021
I. S. Khawaja, T. D. Hurwitz (eds.), *Sleep Disorders in Selected Psychiatric Settings*, https://doi.org/10.1007/978-3-030-59309-4_6

She was anxiously anticipating a promotion and was taking all the required trainings for her new role. Her work requires her to travel to Europe and Asia once a month for a week at a time. She completed her international trips in the first trimester of her pregnancy as she did not want to travel in her last trimester. She used melatonin 5 mg and zolpidem CR 6.25 mg in the past to adjust to different time zones. She did not take any medications during pregnancy due to potential risks to the baby.

Examination/Mental Status Exam BP 116/72, pulse 81/min, temp 36.7 °C (98 °F), respiratory rate 22, height 5′ 5.5″ (1.664 m), weight 218 lbs. (98.9 kg), SpO$_2$ 99%. Body mass index (BMI) is 35.73 kg/m^2. The general and neurological exams were normal.

Special Studies

Actigraphy

Polysomnogram

Results

Actigraphy study (Fig. 6.1) was done for two consecutive weeks of which the first was a work week and the second was a vacation week. It showed a variable bedtime ranging from 11:00 PM to 3:00 AM and wake-up time ranging from 8:00 AM to noon. Some sleep fragmentation and arousals at night were observed; there were no periods of prolonged wakefulness at night.

Overnight polysomnogram (Fig. 6.2) showed a decreased sleep efficiency of 79%, excessive sleep fragmentation with an arousal index of 15/hour, and a wake after sleep onset period of 65 min (AHI 4.6, REM AHI 12.2). There was no evidence of significant hypoxemia. Periodic limb movements were not observed.

Question: What Is the Diagnosis? What Would You Recommend to Improve Sleep Quality?

Differential Diagnosis and Diagnosis

This patient presented with insomnia associated with pregnancy and situational anxiety. Her history revealed occasional mild snoring; however, polysomnogram did not

Fig. 6.1 shows two consecutive weeks of recording. Sleep time is indicated at the top of the graph. Sleep phase is indicated by the shaded area. (This image is original and has not been printed online or in paper in the past.)

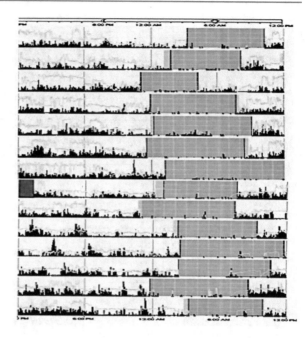

show clinically significant obstructive sleep apnea. She had travelled across time zones suggesting a jet lag-related sleep disorder, and her poor sleep hygiene further worsened her insomnia. The differential diagnosis also included delayed sleep phase circadian rhythm disorder and paradoxical insomnia. There was absence of excessive daytime sleepiness suggesting hyperarousal, and her impaired functioning was limited to the very early morning, both of which made an uncomplicated delayed sleep wake phase disorder far less likely than an insomnia of pregnancy.

General Remarks

Insomnia is characterized by difficulty initiating and maintaining sleep with impairments of daytime functioning. Insomnia may present as a primary disorder or as a symptom of other medical disorders like anxiety, depression, medication side effects, adjustment disorder, and other sleep-related disorders. It is reported as a symptom of obstructive sleep apnea, snoring, circadian rhythm disorders, shift work disorders, movement disorders, and parasomnias. The criteria for diagnosis are difficulty falling asleep, difficulty staying asleep, or early awakening despite the opportunity for sleep. Symptoms must be associated with impaired daytime functioning and occur at least three times per week for at least 1 month [3]. Although insomnia is more commonly found and reported by women, it is underreported and underdiagnosed in pregnancy as the associated symptoms of nocturia, acid reflux, and restlessness are attributed to disturbed sleep.

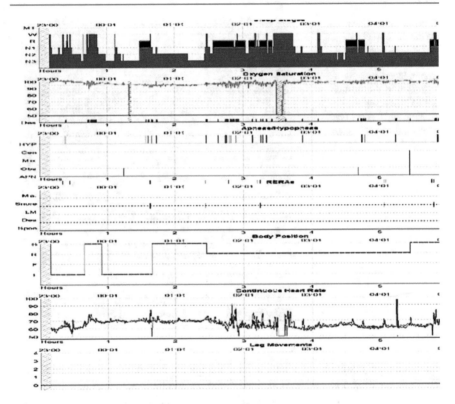

Fig. 6.2 shows an overnight polysomnography significant for excessive sleep fragmentation, few obstructive hypopneas, and respiratory effort-related arousals. (This image is original and has not been printed online or in paper in the past.)

The 3-P model, also known as Spielman model, defines the predisposing, precipitating, and perpetuating factors as an assessment tool for insomnia guiding treatment and behavior changes required to successfully treat the disorder. In this particular patient, the predisposing factors are the state of pregnancy with elevated hormone levels and her tendency to worry. The precipitating factors are the stressful events triggering the onset of her symptoms. This patient had a stressful job situation anticipating promotion and completing the required training and travel associated with obtaining that promotion. The perpetuating factors are her maladaptive coping skills including her poor sleep hygiene. The target of successful treatment is developing the skills for overcoming the precipitating factors and making behavioral changes to reduce the perpetuating factors. A detailed history, an assessment, and a definition of realistic goals are the key to treatment success. Tools like sleep diaries, actigraphy, and polysomnography to evaluate for comorbid sleep disorders can facilitate diagnosis and guide treatment.

Treatment includes behavioral, psychological, and pharmacological interventions, in addition to the various complementary and alternative treatments that most patients try before approaching a clinician. Non-pharmacologic therapies include sleep hygiene techniques, cognitive behavioral therapy for insomnia, relaxation therapy, multicomponent therapy, and paradoxical intention. Sleep restriction, avoidance of excessive time spent in bed, and setting a strict expectation for time in and out of bed improve sleep latency and sleep maintenance through strengthening homeostatic sleep drive. Reducing the bedtime dread associated with struggling to fall asleep and false beliefs about sleep are helped by increased homeostatic drive by restricting time in bed and providing supportive counseling. Sleep restriction also switches the patient's focus from trying to fall asleep to staying awake. Stimulus control involves going to bed only when sleepy, arising when unable to sleep after 20 minutes in bed, avoiding daytime naps, and stimulating behavior like eating in bed, watching TV or reading from an electronic device in bed or just prior to bedtime, and strictly keeping a scheduled wake-up time.

Pharmacologic treatments during pregnancy may be considered if clinically indicated to avoid adverse pregnancy outcomes including postpartum depression. Management of anxiety, depression, and other comorbid conditions will generally improve sleep complaints. The risks of pharmacotherapy must be weighed against their benefits due to the possible risk of teratogenicity associated with some medications [1]. Most sedative hypnotic drugs commonly used for insomnia are pregnancy category C, D, or X [2]; therefore, cognitive behavioral therapy for insomnia in combination with sleep restriction and setting a realistic expectation of sleep has safer outcomes than medication. Antihistamines considered safe in pregnancy may be used for cases not responding to CBT-I [1].

Pearls/Take-Home Points
- Insomnia is a common, although underdiagnosed sleep complaint, during pregnancy affecting quality of life and pregnancy outcomes for this population of women.
- Identification of predisposing, precipitating, and perpetuating factors for insomnia in individual patients guides behavior and treatment intervention.
- Pharmacologic management of insomnia is indicated in patients with significant limitation of daytime functioning and patients with comorbid disorders.

Suggested Reading

1. Hashmi AM, Bhatia SK, Bhatia SK, Khawaja IS. Insomnia during pregnancy: diagnosis and rational interventions. Pak J Med Sci. 2016;32(4):1030–7.
2. Jones CR. Diagnostic and management approach to common sleep disorders during pregnancy. Clin Obstet Gynecol. 2013;56(2):360–71.
3. Maness DL, Khan M. Nonpharmacologic Management of Chronic Insomnia. Am Fam Physician. 2015;92(12):1058–64.
4. Dørheim SK, Bjorvatn B, Eberhard-Gran M. Can insomnia in pregnancy predict postpartum depression? A longitudinal, population-based study. PLoS One. 2014;9(4):e94674. Published 2014 Apr 14. https://doi.org/10.1371/journal.pone.0094674.

Obstructive Sleep Apnea in Pregnancy

7

Safia S. Khan and Gregory S. Carter

Clinical History/Case

Miss N.C. was a 27-year-old G3P2A0 woman at 14 weeks' gestational age who was referred to the sleep clinic for suspected obstructive sleep apnea. Her pregnancy had been complicated by hypertension. She had a history of an emergency C-section due to pre-eclampsia and fetal distress at 39 weeks of gestation. Following general anesthesia, she could not be extubated for 24 hours due to significant hypoxemia. Her husband reported a history of continuous loud snoring for the 5 years they have been together associated with intermittent arousals and witnessed apneas that had worsened during her previous pregnancy 2 years ago. The arousals were brief, and she was able to return to sleep in less than 5 minutes. She reported taking a nap daily after lunch and complained of excessive daytime sleepiness despite sleeping an average of 9 hours a night. She had been obese since childhood despite multiple dieting attempts without significant improvement. Her medications included prenatal multivitamins, ferrous sulfate, and labetalol.

S. S. Khan (✉)
Department of Family and Community Medicine, Department of Neurology and Neurotherapeutics at University of Texas Southwestern Medical Center, Dallas, TX, USA

Parkland Sleep Center, Parkland Medical Hospital, Dallas, TX, USA

Texas Health Resources Presbyterian Hospital, Dallas, TX, USA
e-mail: Safia.khan@utsouthwestern.edu

G. S. Carter
UT Southwestern Sleep Medicine Fellowship Program, Department of Neurology and Neurotherapeutics at The University of Texas Southwestern Medical Center at Dallas, Dallas, TX, USA
e-mail: Gregory.carter@utsouthwestern.edu

© Springer Nature Switzerland AG 2021
I. S. Khawaja, T. D. Hurwitz (eds.), *Sleep Disorders in Selected Psychiatric Settings*, https://doi.org/10.1007/978-3-030-59309-4_7

Examination/Mental Status Exam

Her physical exam showed the following: BP 123/67, pulse 94, temp 36.3 °C (97.4 °F), height 5′ 5″ (1.651 m), weight 368 lbs. (166.9 kg), SpO_2 100%, BMI 61.24 kg/m². Her oropharyngeal exam showed a crowded airway with large tongue and short anteroposterior diameter of oropharynx, Mallampati: IV, a neck circumference of 19 inches, and normal neurologic exam.

Question 1 Given the above symptoms, what is the best treatment option for this patient?

A. Tracheostomy
B. Maternal weight loss
C. Avoidance of supine sleeping position
D. Treatment with CPAP
E. Mandibular advancement device

Question 2 What is the possible outcome in this patient with untreated disease?

A. Gestational diabetes
B. Hypertension
C. Pre-eclampsia
D. Intrauterine growth retardation
E. All of the above

Special Studies

She received a nocturnal in-laboratory attended diagnostic polysomnography (shown in Figs. 7.1 and 7.2)

Polysomnography

Results

In-lab polysomnography (Fig. 7.1) with split night protocol was done which showed severe obstructive sleep apnea with an Apnea hypopnea index (AHI) of 110/hour, associated with significant hypoxemia (SPO_2 below 88% for 21 minutes, nadir SPO_2 of 62%) (Fig. 7.2). Sleep was fragmented with an arousal index of 108/hour.

Optimal treatment pressure was determined to be 8 cm water, AHI was zero at this pressure, and supine REM was not achieved at this pressure.

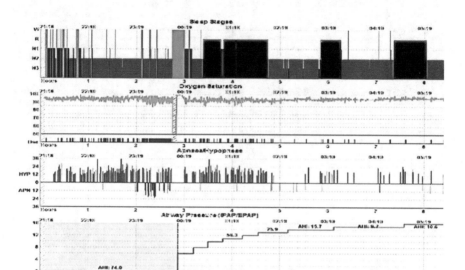

Fig. 7.1 An entire night polysomnogram plot showing sleep stages, oxygen desaturation, respiratory events, respiratory effort-related arousals, positive airway pressure, and body position. (I certify this picture is original and has not been printed in print or online in the past)

Transcutaneous CO_2 at the start of the polysomnography was 43 mm Hg, and at the end of the sleep study, it was 45 mm Hg.

Differential Diagnosis and Diagnosis

This patient had a significant history of loud snoring and witnessed apneas in the setting of morbid obesity and a prior history of prenatal and postnatal complications. She had prolonged recovery from anesthesia due to significant hypoxemia. This was unlikely to be due to simple snoring and upper airway resistance syndrome as these do not lead to significant hypoxemia. There was no evidence of central apneas, and transcutaneous CO_2 levels were less than 50 mm Hg; therefore, the diagnosis of obesity hypoventilation could be ruled out. This patient had severe obstructive sleep apnea associated with significant hypoxemia leading to excessive daytime sleepiness and tiredness despite sleeping an adequate number of hours each night and taking a nap during the day.

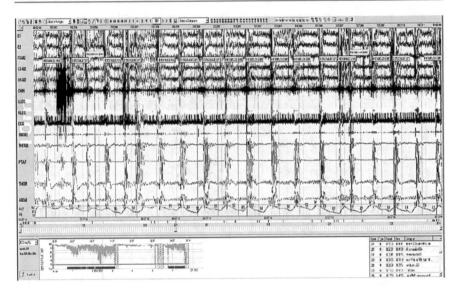

Fig. 7.2 Ten-minute tracing during REM and NREM sleep showing obstructive apneas, arousals, and snoring. (I certify this picture is original and has not been printed in print or online in the past)

General Remarks

Pregnancy is a dynamic process with significant hormonal changes leading to physical and physiologic changes in the expectant mother. Obstructive sleep apnea (OSA), while commonly diagnosed in obese men and women, is often underdiagnosed in pregnant women. Snoring, witnessed apneas, excessive daytime sleepiness, and fatigue are common symptoms of OSA [1]. These symptoms overlap with normal physiologic changes in pregnancy. Many women experience reduced quality of sleep, reduced sleep efficiency, increasing arousals due to acid reflux, fetal movements, nocturia, and pressure on the urinary bladder as the pregnancy progresses [1].

Pregnancy is associated with features protective against OSA and added risks for pregnancy-related OSA. Protective features include reduction in REM sleep stage, tendency to avoid supine sleeping position, possible estrogen-related reduction in AHI, progesterone-induced activity of pharyngeal dilator muscles, and progesterone-driven increase in respiratory drive.

Risk factors for pregnancy-onset sleep-disordered breathing (SDB) include estrogen-mediated nasopharyngeal edema, hyperemia, and vasomotor rhinitis, which decrease nasopharyngeal patency and increase airflow resistance. Other factors worsening OSA in pregnancy are weight gain, commonly up to 20% of body weight over the course of pregnancy, decreased functional residual capacity (FRC) secondary to upward displacement of the diaphragm, and decreased oxygen reserve secondary to increased oxygen consumption and decreased FRC [1].

Treatment of OSA in pregnancy includes limiting weight gain, avoiding the supine sleeping position, head elevation while sleeping, and restriction of sedative/hypnotics. Continuous positive airway pressure is the treatment of choice in pregnant women with moderate to severe OSA. Tracheostomy would be reserved for extreme circumstances with severe pulmonary hypertension. Mandibular advancement devices require custom fitting and production time and may not be as useful within the time limits of pregnancy.

Complications of untreated OSA in pregnancy include gestational diabetes, gestational hypertension, pre-eclampsia, and intrauterine growth retardation [2–5]. These outcomes are mediated in part by intermittent hypoxia-reoxygenation, which may lead to increased sympathetic activity, oxidative stress, and inflammation. During pregnancy, these disturbances contribute to maternal cardio-metabolic derangements such as gestational hypertension, diabetes, and pre-eclampsia [2–5]. An increased association of maternal obstructive sleep apnea and an increased risk of in-hospital death, pulmonary embolism, and cardiomyopathy were noted by Louis et al. in a large database of 55 million delivery-related hospital discharges [5]. This relationship persisted and was exacerbated in the presence of obesity. Pregnant women with obstructive sleep apnea have a higher rate of cesarean births, neonatal prematurity, and respiratory complications.

Pearls/Take-Home Points
- There is a strong association of obesity and obstructive sleep apnea in pregnancy; adequate weight monitoring can prevent adverse outcomes associated with untreated OSA.
- While excessive sleepiness, tiredness, and snoring can be normal in pregnancy, evaluation for obstructive sleep apnea should be considered in the presence of obesity, hypertension, excessive weight gain, pre-eclampsia, and delayed intrauterine fetal development, plus complications during delivery and/or prolonged recovery from anesthesia [5].
- Treatment of OSA with CPAP is recommended for women with moderate to severe OSA, and conservative management may be considered for women with mild disease.
- An evaluation of OSA after delivery is indicated in cases of adverse pregnancy outcomes in association with obesity, gestational hypertension, gestational diabetes mellitus, and pre-eclampsia.

Suggested Readings (References)

1. Longworth H, et al. Screening methods for obstructive sleep apnoea in severely obese pregnant women. Clin Obes. 2017;7:239–44.
2. Bourjeily G, et al. Obstructive sleep apnea in pregnancy is associated with adverse maternal outcomes: a national cohort. Sleep Med. 2017;38:50–7. https://doi.org/10.1016/j.sleep.2017.06.035. Epub 2017 Jul 26.

3. Pamidi S, Pinto L, Marc I, et al. Maternal sleep-disordered breathing and adverse pregnancy outcomes: a systematic review and metaanalysis. Am J Obstet Gynecol. 2014;210:52e1–14.
4. Cain MA, Louis JM. Sleep disordered breathing and adverse pregnancy outcomes. Clin Lab Med. 2016;36:435–46. https://doi.org/10.1016/j.cll.2016.01.001.
5. Louis JM, et al. Obstructive sleep apnea and severe maternal-infant morbidity/mortality in the United States, 1998-2009. Sleep. 2014;37(5):843–9. https://doi.org/10.5665/sleep.3644.

Management of Restless Legs in Pregnancy: An Obstetrician, Internal Medicine Physician, and Perinatal Psychiatrist Work Together in an Obstetric Clinic

8

Felice Watt, Alison Uku, and Adam S. Akers

Obstetrician

History

Mrs. Ardis is a 29-year Caucasian woman in her third pregnancy, having delivered two previous children, who presented to the antenatal clinic at 28 weeks' gestation.

Her first pregnancy at age 25 resulted in forceps-assisted vaginal birth with episiotomy repair and more than average blood loss. Her recovery was slow, complicated by perineal discomfort, and she required antibiotics for a perineal wound infection, which caused a prolonged healing time.

Her second pregnancy a year later was straightforward except for the occasional sensation of tingling and crawling sensation in her legs, which began at 24 weeks and gradually worsened through her third trimester. She requested an elective birth by cesarean section due to anxiety and her traumatic experience in the first birth. This was performed at 39 weeks, also resulting in slightly more than average blood loss. She had an uncomplicated postpartum period.

The current pregnancy was unplanned, as she was unable to keep her gynecology appointment to discuss contraceptive options. The pregnancy interval was 1 year, and she was anxious about this pregnancy.

At presentation, she described a 2-month history of the itchy, crawling sensation in her legs that she had in her previous pregnancy. She also had an uncontrollable

F. Watt (✉)
Department of Psychiatry, Sidra Medicine, Doha, Qatar
e-mail: fwatt@sidra.org

A. Uku
Department of Obstetrics and Gynecology, Sidra Medicine, Doha, Qatar

A. S. Akers
Department of Internal Medicine, Sidra Medicine, Doha, Qatar

© Springer Nature Switzerland AG 2021
I. S. Khawaja, T. D. Hurwitz (eds.), *Sleep Disorders in Selected Psychiatric Settings*, https://doi.org/10.1007/978-3-030-59309-4_8

urge to move her legs, particularly at night, making it difficult for her to sleep despite using emollient creams and ointments and antihistamines, which only seemed to give temporary relief of her symptoms. Her anxiety was made more evident by her fatigue, and she feared that she might need to go back on the medication that she had taken as a teenager to "calm her nerves."

She had no other significant past medical or drug history. She did not report leg cramps. She was not taking any medications except for pregnancy vitamins and occasional diphenhydramine 25 mg at night and had no known allergies.

She attained menarche at age 12 and had regular though moderately heavy periods each month for 7 days for which she would take the occasional analgesic. There was no history suggestive of sexually transmitted infections, and her Pap smears were normal and up to date.

She was a nonsmoker and drank about six units of alcohol per week before pregnancy, none since being pregnant.

Her father is hypertensive on medication, while her mother is on regular antidepressant medication and takes mild sedation for her insomnia. Her mother and older sister also experienced mild burning or itchy sensation in their legs as well and uncontrollable leg movements when trying to sleep in pregnancy. They live abroad.

Mrs. Ardis is a housewife, while her husband, who is a heavy smoker, works 12-hour shifts, including weekends, on a construction site some distance from home.

Physical Examination

General examination revealed a tired-looking, anxious woman whose vital signs were stable. An abdominal examination revealed a gravid uterus appropriate for her gestation and positive fetal heart with an active fetus. There were no leg varicosities or edema.

A review of her routine antenatal screen revealed hemoglobin of 105 g/l (corrected for gestational age of the pregnancy this falls within the normal range); renal function and electrolytes, serology screen, antibody screen, and urinalysis were nil of note.

Provisional Diagnosis

Normal pregnancy
  Mild anxiety and family history of mental health problems
  Possible restless legs syndrome (RLS)

Management Plan

1. Iron studies, vitamin D, folate, and B12 were ordered, given Mrs. Ardis' history and experience of tiredness.

2. Referral to sleep medicine for further evaluation of possible restless legs syndrome.
3. Referral to the perinatal mental health team for assessment and management of anxiety.
4. Normal antenatal care.
5. Arrange a multidisciplinary team meeting with internal medicine and perinatal psychiatry before her next appointment in 4 weeks.

Sleep Medicine Physician

The sleep medicine physician reviewed Mrs. Ardis' history and agreed with the provisional diagnosis of RLS. He asked her to complete the Restless Legs Syndrome Rating Scale [1] and a severity score. She scored "severe" on questions 4 and 5 regarding sleep disturbance and reported "moderate" mood disturbance from her restless legs symptoms – her total score was 23 points (in the severe range), and her self-report severity scale for her symptoms of the previous week was 6 (severe restless legs).

Physical examination was unchanged, and the neurological exam of lower legs was normal.

Iron studies revealed ferritin of 10 µg/L, and her blood smear showed a mild hypochromic microcytic picture consistent with iron deficiency anemia. Vitamin B12, folate, and vitamin D were all normal.

The physician decided not to perform routine polysomnography as there were no indications of other sleep disorders, such as obstructive sleep apnea [2].

The physician discussed his diagnosis and the results with Mrs. Ardis and recommended the following plan.

Management

1. An iron supplement was prescribed – 60 mg elemental iron by mouth daily on an empty stomach.
2. Education regarding the diagnosis of RLS, including the likelihood of resolution straight after delivery. He noted that medications could be helpful in management but advised Mrs. Ardis to try non-pharmacological strategies first, particularly:
    • Reducing potentially activating factors, such as tea and coffee and the sedating antihistamine she had been taking, which had been of no benefit and had possibly made things worse.
    • Regular exercise in keeping with her stage of pregnancy
3. Recheck the ferritin and hemoglobin in 2 weeks to check the response to iron replacement.

Perinatal Psychiatrist

The perinatal psychiatrist saw Mrs. Ardis 2 weeks after her obstetrician referral. The psychiatrist also reviewed her medical record and blood results. Mrs. Ardis described symptoms of mild to moderate anxiety dating from when she realized she was pregnant again. She was worried about how she was going to cope with a third child, especially as she was already exhausted looking after her two young children. She was already ruminating on how this baby would be delivered, given her previous deliveries. She reported tension in her neck and arms. She also described depressive symptoms emerging over the preceding 4 weeks – including reduced enjoyment of her children, crying several times a week, irritability, lack of energy, and negative thoughts about herself (she was blaming herself for not organizing contraception sooner). She described initial insomnia of 1 hour, saying that her legs felt jumpy and restless and she had to keep moving around in the bed to get comfortable. She was then able to fall asleep until her youngest child woke around 5 am. She was still able to enjoy her food, and according to the obstetrician, her weight gain during pregnancy was within the normal range. There was no suicidal ideation or thoughts of harm to others.

Past Psychiatric History

Mrs. Ardis noted that she had been anxious ("worse than I am now") during her last pregnancy, where the focus of her anxiety had been fear of another traumatic birth and long recovery period.

She described feeling low for several months after her first delivery but had not sought help.

She reported being anxious for about 6 months leading up to her final high school exams. Her mother had taken her to a psychiatrist, who prescribed a medication, which she took for a week and then stopped because she was not feeling any better.

Substance Use History

Mrs. Ardis confirmed drinking approximately six standard drinks per week before becoming pregnant, commenting that she had never used to drink this much but found that a glass of wine at night helped her to "get through the evening with the kids."

Family History

Mrs. Ardis' mother had always suffered from depression and had taken medication (she was not sure what) for years. Although her father was hypertensive now, he had always been very healthy.

She described a close family and a happy upbringing, although she said her mother tended to be overprotective and a worrier. Mrs. Ardis is the younger of two sisters. Her sister had three children and had also experienced "jumping legs" during two of her pregnancies, and her mother recalled having the same difficulties when she was pregnant with her daughters. Neither had experienced this problem apart from during their pregnancies.

Social History

Mrs. Ardis had completed high school and trained in office administration. She had worked for the same company until her marriage to Mr. Ardis 6 years ago. Soon after their marriage, he was transferred to the Middle East, and the couple has continued to reside there. Although Mrs. Ardis had made some local friends, she missed her family terribly and found it difficult when her husband had to travel for work. He works long hours but helps her with the children when he is home.

Mental State Examination

Mrs. Ardis arrived late with her youngest child, who played happily with some toys in the room, from time to time, bringing them to his mum to admire. She looked tired and worried, but rapport was quickly established, with her commenting that she was grateful to have someone to talk to about how she was feeling. There was no abnormal behavior. She described her mood as low; her affect was predominantly anxious, and she cried briefly when describing her shock at discovering she was pregnant again. She went on to smile, briefly, saying that now she had got used to the idea, she was looking forward to meeting her next little one. She described worry thoughts about the delivery, her ability to cope with three children once the baby was born, and her parents' health. There were no psychotic features, and she was cognitively intact. There was no evidence of current risk to herself or others. She was keen to engage in treatment.

Formulation

Mrs. Ardis described symptoms of moderate antenatal depression and anxiety. She has a history of anxiety as a teenager during exams and in her second pregnancy after the traumatic birth of her first child. She had possibly experienced an unrecognized depressive episode after her first child. There was a family history of depression and anxiety in her mother. Lack of social support and separation from her family, as well as the demands of looking after two young children, were significant exacerbating factors. Initial insomnia associated with her RLS was likely to be impacting on her mood.

Management

The psychiatrist ordered thyroid function tests in case abnormal thyroid function was contributing to Mrs. Ardis' anxiety and depression.

She shared her formulation with Mrs. Ardis and discussed management options. It was essential to consider the impact of symptoms, not only on her well-being, but also on the developing fetus, the pregnancy, and her capacity to care for her young family in her current social context.

The treatment discussion included consideration of both psychological and pharmacological interventions, and potential impacts on the fetus and her pregnancy were discussed. Mrs. Ardis was keen to pursue psychological therapy, particularly as she had not liked the medication she tried as a teenager. Cognitive behavioral therapy (CBT) was recommended, with particular focuses of the therapy to be a reduction of her depressive and anxiety symptomatology and improvement in her sleep.

Mrs. Ardis agreed to see the perinatal clinical psychologist, and a psychiatrist review appointment was arranged for 4 weeks.

Multidisciplinary Team Meeting

The obstetrician, sleep medicine physician, psychiatrist, and psychologist met briefly at the antenatal clinic before Mrs. Ardis' next obstetric appointment to review her case, discuss progress, and consider ongoing treatment plans.

By now, Mrs. Ardis was in her 33rd week of pregnancy. Her thyroid function tests had come back as within the normal range for her stage of pregnancy.

The psychologist indicated that Mrs. Ardis' mood and anxiety had improved after three sessions of CBT. She had incorporated sleep hygiene strategies into her daily routine, but unfortunately, she was still taking about an hour to get off to sleep, stating that her restless legs made it difficult for her to settle. The psychologist indicated that Mrs. Ardis was attending a pregnancy yoga class every week and was walking for half an hour most evenings with a mother she had met at her yoga class, while her husband looked after the children.

The psychologist indicated she would continue CBT with Mrs. Ardis, noting that her anxiety might increase as delivery approached. The emerging evidence regarding the potential impact of disturbed sleep [3] and RLS [4] on pregnancy outcomes and fetal well-being was discussed by the team. The psychiatrist said she would discuss pharmacological options for treatment of her restless legs and associated sleep disturbance with Mrs. Ardis at her upcoming appointment the following week.

The obstetrician indicted that routine obstetric care would continue as indicated, and she hoped that Mrs. Ardis would be willing to try a vaginal birth after cesarean section (VBAC) as her postpartum recovery would be quicker.

Her repeat iron studies showed hemoglobin of 110 g/l, and ferritin increased to 25 µg/L, indicating a response to the iron supplementation.

Progress

Mrs. Ardis' pregnancy continued with no unforeseen difficulties.

At her psychiatrist review, she presented as less depressed and anxious and indicated that she was finding her CBT sessions very helpful. She was relieved that her mother was coming to stay with the family for 6 weeks after the baby's birth. Mrs. Ardis stated that she felt confident in her obstetrician's advice and support and that she would like to attempt a VBAC as recommended. Unfortunately, she was still troubled by her restless legs, and on some evenings, it took her 2 hours to get off to sleep, leaving her feeling exhausted the next day. She had cut out tea and coffee from her diet, was no longer taking the antihistamine, and was compliant with her iron supplementation. She was continuing with pregnancy yoga and her regular walks.

The psychiatrist discussed the option of medication for the treatment of her insomnia/restless legs, acknowledging that Mrs. Ardis had previously said she would prefer not to take medication. She recommended that clonazepam 0.5 mg at night would be the most helpful medication to take at this stage and went on to describe how, when considering taking medication during pregnancy, it was important to weigh up the risks and benefits of taking the medication for both the woman and her baby. The psychiatrist described how there was increasing evidence that sleep deprivation [3] (as well as anxiety and depression [5, 6]) could impact on obstetric outcomes and that although it was very encouraging that her depression and anxiety had improved, her restless legs and associated insomnia were a persisting problem, not only for her, but potentially for her pregnancy and baby's wellbeing [3]. She then went on to outline the particular risks associated with clonazepam, explaining that the baseline risk for fetal abnormalities is 2–3% [7]; as her baby was at 34 weeks gestation, the period of organ formation was finished, and so there was no risk of major fetal abnormalities being caused by the clonazepam. The potential that medications taken during later pregnancy could impact on the baby's developing nervous system was discussed; of the few studies done on long-term impacts of babies exposed to benzodiazepines during pregnancy, several have been reassuring [8, 9]. One study [10] suggests a small increase in fearfulness and social withdrawal in children exposed. There are potential difficulties of development of tolerance and dependence for the mother and the baby, a very slight increased need for respiratory support at birth, and monitoring of the baby for any signs of withdrawal. On the dose of medication prescribed, the risk of these problems was low. The psychiatrist undertook, however, to consult with neonatology colleagues, who would arrange to be present at the birth. The nursing staff would monitor the baby for any withdrawal symptoms.

Mrs. Ardis said she would like to take clonazepam 0.5 mg only on nights when she felt she needed it. She would like a prescription but would discuss it with her husband before starting. Her psychiatrist gave her some printed information about clonazepam during pregnancy (Mother to Baby Fact Sheet) [11].

Outcome

Mrs. Ardis spoke with her husband, and they decided she would take clonazepam 0.5 mg on nights when he was at home so that he could attend to the children if they woke at night, if she was too sleepy to do so. At her following psychiatrist appointment, she reported that she was taking clonazepam 0.5 mg approximately three times a week. After taking clonazepam, her legs would feel more relaxed, and she would be asleep within about 40 minutes; she recounted that knowing that she would experience some relief had lessened her feelings of anxiety. Although her pregnancy was advancing, she did not feel as tired in the day and was more able to cope with parenting her children and getting ready for the impending birth. She had reduced her CBT sessions to fortnightly, and the improvement in her depressive and anxiety symptoms was maintained. Mrs. Ardis was advised to try to minimize clonazepam use in the week before her expected delivery to reduce the possibility of neonatal withdrawal [12].

Mrs. Ardis went into labor spontaneously at 39 weeks and delivered a healthy baby girl. A neonatologist was present at delivery; however, no respiratory assistance was required. Her baby established breastfeeding well and did not show evidence of withdrawal symptoms.

At her 6-week postnatal review, Mrs. Ardis reported that her RLS had stopped soon after delivery and that further clonazepam was not needed. She reported a good birth experience, had bonded well with baby Jane, and was grateful for her mother's support. She remained free of depressive and anxiety symptoms. Although her baby was feeding twice a night, she was able to get back to sleep after each feed.

Diagnosis

For pregnancy-related RLS, the same diagnostic criteria as for non-pregnancy RLS are recommended [13]:

1. Desire to move the limbs, usually associated with paresthesia/dysesthesias
2. Onset or exacerbation with rest
3. Partial or complete relief by activity
4. Onset or worsening of symptoms during night times

Differential Diagnosis

Pregnancy is a major risk factor for RLS occurring in up to 34% of pregnant women [14]. The odds ratio for the prevalence of RLS increases with parity up to 3.57 with three or more pregnancies [15].

Differential diagnosis includes (can co-occur):

1. Positional discomfort during pregnancy – relieved by position change rather than by recurrent leg movements

2. Nocturnal cramps – sudden, painful tightness, muscle hardness
3. Leg edema
4. Venous stasis
5. Neuropathy (including related to compression and stretch neuropathies) – numbness is not a typical symptom of RLS
6. Sore leg muscles; ligament tenderness or tendon strain

Rarer causes include arthritis, radiculopathy, renal disease, complex regional pain syndrome, drug-induced akathisia (antidepressants, antipsychotics), and sickle cell anemia.

RLS may occur with psychiatric comorbidity, particularly anxiety and depression; these must be screened for as it can affect treatment planning.

Discussion

Restless leg syndrome (RLS) and periodic limb movement disorder (PLMD) are similar and overlapping conditions that have an increased incidence in pregnancy [16]. RLS is a sensorimotor disorder characterized by an irresistible and uncomfortable urge to move the legs, relief with movement, and onset before sleep and at night. The diagnosis is made clinically using the International RLS Study Group (IRLSSG) Score [13].The incidence of RLS in the general population is approximately 5–15%, and the incidence in pregnancy is higher at 10–34% [14]. The strongest risk factors are a personal (either during previous pregnancies or while not pregnant) and family history of the disorder, as well as parity [13, 17]. A positive family history of RLS is reported in up to 92% of patients [18]. The fact that the incidence of RLS is identical in men and nulliparous women suggests that the excess incidence in women is related solely to parity [15, 19, 20]. Many of the studies on the incidence and severity of RLS rely on survey and retrospective data. In one carefully designed and executed prospective study in Zurich, Switzerland, the incidence of RLS in pregnancy was lower than generally stated (12%), and these patients had an earlier onset of symptoms (59% before 20 weeks' gestation). This study used the IRLSS for diagnosis and leg actigraphy to measure the severity of periodic leg movements. A personal and family history of RLS, as well as smoking, were risk factors, but not an iron deficiency, estrogen levels, or leg circumference (a measure of water retention) [21].

Some authors divide RLS into primary idiopathic and secondary types (related to weight gain in pregnancy, iron deficiency, folate deficiency, vitamin D deficiency, neuropathy, end-stage renal disease, Parkinson's disease, rheumatoid arthritis, and fibromyalgia) [22]. However, the data on these secondary causes of RLS in pregnancy are sparse and conflicting [23, 24]. Most evidence points to pregnancy as an exacerbating factor in genetically vulnerable women rather than a cause of RLS in and of itself because of the strong association with family history and a relatively high recurrence rate after pregnancy [25]. Also, RLS symptoms often do not respond to the treatment of these secondary causes raising the question of causation or mere association.

There is a peak in the incidence of RLS in the third trimester, and the disorder generally remits after delivery [26–29]. Therefore, it is tempting to invoke estrogen levels as the cause of RLS in pregnancy, since they also peak in the third trimester and fall precipitously after delivery. Also, estrogen is known to affect dopamine levels in the striatonigral system [30]. However, clinical studies are mixed as to the association, and less than one-third of women develop RLS in pregnancy despite these high levels. Even less evidence exists for the association between RLS and other hormones such as progestin, prolactin, and thyroid hormone [31].

Iron and folate are integral in the production of dopamine in the brain and, therefore, could play a role in the pathogenesis of RLS in pregnancy. Iron is a cofactor for tyrosine hydroxylase, and folate is involved in the recycling of tetrahydrobiopterin [32]. There are several reports of an association between iron deficiency anemia and RLS [33], and some show no association [34]; however, interventional studies are mixed, and it is not clear that treating iron deficiency improves the symptoms of RLS [35–37]. Since RLS resolves rapidly after delivery and iron levels are slow to recover, it seems unlikely that iron deficiency is a viable cause of RLS in pregnancy.

Variants in five genes are associated with RLS: MEIS1, BTBD9, MAP2K5, LBXCOR1, and PTPRD [38].The first three genetic variants may account for up to 50% of cases of RLS [39, 40]. The MEIS1 gene may be involved in limb development, indicating that RLS may be, in part, a developmental disorder.

Symptoms can range from mild to very severe, as measured by the IRLSSG rating scale [1].

In nonpregnant patients, RLS has been definitively linked to a disturbance in sleep through a questionnaire, interview, and polysomnographic studies [41]. Severe RLS in pregnancy is thought to disrupt subjective sleep quality and daytime functional status, as evidenced by survey data [42, 43, 44, 45]. However, since pregnancy itself can cause sleep disturbance, high-quality data for this claim is difficult to find. One small but well-designed polysomnographic study showed no difference in sleep quality scores (Pittsburgh Sleep Quality Index, PSQI) or polysomnographic indices between RLS and non-RLS pregnant patients despite a higher degree of periodic limb movement in the former group [31]. Another small study showed significantly delayed sleep and REM latency in the pregnant RLS group compared to the pregnant non-RLS group [42].

Although sleep deprivation in general has been linked to specific adverse pregnancy outcomes such as preeclampsia, increased rate of cesarean section, preterm delivery, hypertension, and cardiovascular disease [46], a direct link between RLS and these adverse outcomes has not been consistently demonstrated [47].The association of RLS in pregnancy with hypertension and cardiovascular disease is inconsistent. In a small study, depression, as measured by the Profile of Mood States (POMS), was statistically more significant in the RLS group than the non-RLS group (POMS 1.6.vs 0.14, $p = 0.012$) [42].

There is no evidence that RLS increases the risk of fetal malformations.

Restless legs syndrome in pregnancy can be confused with and coexist with other limb disorders such as periodic limb movement of sleep (PLMS), nocturnal leg cramps, stretch or compression neuropathies, and edema. Nocturnal leg cramps occur at about the same rate as RLS in pregnancy and are muscle pains in the calves, which are relieved with stretching.

Management

RLS treatment should be individualized, considering symptom severity, comorbidities, and the woman's situation and preferences.

Education of the woman about the usual course of restless legs in pregnancy is often helpful, providing hope that the symptoms will most likely reduce or disappear after delivery. Advice and assistance should be provided to help the woman address possible exacerbating factors including nicotine, caffeine consumption, irregular sleep, insufficient sleep, sedating antihistamines, antidepressants, dopaminergic agents, and anti-emetics, which may be used to treat pregnancy nausea [13]. Management of obstructive sleep apnea, if present, can also be helpful. Good sleep hygiene can help prevent the development of insomnia related to RLS [2].

Iron and any other vitamin deficiencies should be treated.

Non-pharmacological strategies are first-line treatments and have varying success in reducing symptoms (noting that there is a significant placebo response). Moderate physical exercise in the absence of contraindications has been shown to increase deep sleep, improve RLS, and benefit mental health [48]. Interventions with a reasonable evidence base include yoga and pneumatic pressure devices and massage [13].

Women with severe symptoms unresponsive to non-pharmacological-pharmacological strategies may benefit from pharmacological intervention. Many of the first-line drugs for the treatment of RLS have minimal safety data in pregnancy [47]. The decision to use psychotropic medication during pregnancy may be difficult for the woman and her husband or the prescribing clinician; however for some women, medication will be an important therapeutic option [49]. The decision to treat follows an informed consent process, assisting the woman to weigh up treatment risks and benefits, considering potential impacts of the medication on the woman, her fetus, and pregnancy outcomes as well as the risks of no treatment to the woman, her fetus, and the pregnancy [50]. Potential impacts on the fetus will be influenced by the stage of pregnancy during which treatment is provided and in the newborn by the passage of medications through breast milk in the breastfeeding mother.

Prescribing during pregnancy is guided by fundamental principles, including prescribing medication with lower-risk profiles for the mother and fetus, prescribing at the lowest effective dose needed to achieve a therapeutic response, and regularly reviewing the need for and response to treatment [51].

Clonazepam (0.25–1 mg at night) has one of the more favorable risk/benefit profiles for the treatment of RLS during pregnancy [52]. Although benzodiazepines have been used for more than 40 years, many of the published studies have varying limitations. In terms of the literature regarding clonazepam exposure during pregnancy, findings are often generalized to benzodiazepines in general, rather than to clonazepam in particular, and a number of the studies reporting neonatal outcomes after antenatal exposure are poorly controlled for confounding variables particularly indication for benzodiazepine use, nature and severity of any the maternal illness being treated, a consideration of comorbidities, and the impacts of multiple medications. Nevertheless, a consideration of the nature of the available evidence and the woman's particular situation can assist a woman and her health-care provider.

Although benzodiazepines have previously been reported being associated with an increased risk of congenital abnormalities, particularly or facial clefts [53] later studies have not confirmed this [54]. Possible neurodevelopment impacts due to second and third trimester fetal exposure have been reported. A recent prospective registry analysis [55] found that infants exposed to benzodiazepines during pregnancy had an increased risk of small head circumference compared to unexposed infants; however, the authors noted that this outcome was rare and should be interpreted with caution. A limited number of studies have found an increased risk of low Apgar scores, respiratory distress, preterm birth, and low birth weight in women who filled a prescription of benzodiazepines in the second or third trimester [56, 57]. A separate investigator reported similar findings after pregnancy exposure, including increased rates of admission to the neonatal intensive care unit (NICU) [58]. Neonatal withdrawal symptoms have also been associated with the use of benzodiazepines; usually infants who develop withdrawal symptoms will recover without any lasting sequelae [59]. The syndrome is best minimized by gradually taping the benzodiazepine dose before delivery and ideally should be discontinued at least one week before delivery [59]. In view of this literature, it is recommended that there must be availability of respiratory support/neonatology review at delivery. Only small amounts of clonazepam pass into breast milk [60] and are unlikely to pose a risk to the infant; however, nocturnal sedation in a feeding mother may hamper the capacity to attend to the infant at night, posing potential risks. Co-sleeping with the infant should be avoided as should taking other potentially sedating agents (including alcohol).

Carbidopa-levodopa has been prescribed for RLS in pregnancy for a small number of women without significant adverse outcome [61]; however a potential risk includes augmentation of RLS (an increase in RLS symptom severity [62]).

Low-dose oxycodone (contraindicated in breastfeeding women) is considered a reasonable option for severe symptoms, unresponsive to other interventions after the first trimester of pregnancy [13]. Potential impacts that need to be considered include neonatal abstinence syndrome, dependence, and escalation of the dose in the mother (has not been reported in long-term treatment for RLS) [63, 64].

Although treatment of RLS may improve anxiety and depressive symptoms, specific treatment of depression is required if a depressive disorder is present. Non-pharmacological treatments for mild-moderate depression in pregnancy are recommended; however if pharmacotherapy is required, it is important to note that serotonergic agents, which are usually first-line medications, may worsen RLS [65]. Given this, bupropion, which does not alter the reuptake of serotonin or norepinephrine, is a reasonable option but of course must be prescribed following exploration of the risk/benefit equation during pregnancy and lactation.

Pearls

1. Accurate diagnosis, including consideration of differential diagnosis and associated comorbidities (including medical, other sleep disorders, and psychiatric conditions), is essential.
2. Women with ferritin less than 75 µg/L are likely to benefit from iron replacement.
3. Treatment decisions should be based on symptom severity (including the level of distress and impact) and a consideration of the risk/benefit equation for women and her fetus as part of an informed consent process.
4. Non-pharmacological treatments are the first line.
5. If medications are prescribed, these should be at the lowest effective dose and only as clinically required, with regular reassessment of symptom severity during pregnancy and after delivery.

References

1. International Restless Legs Syndrome Study Group. Validation of the International Restless Legs Syndrome Study Group Rating Scale for restless legs syndrome. Sleep Med. 2003;4(2):121–32.
2. Burman D. Sleep disorders: restless legs syndrome. FP Essentials. 2017;460:29–32.
3. Palagini L, Gemignani A, Bantia S, Manconic M, Mauria M, Riemannd D. Chronic sleep loss during pregnancy as a determinant of stress: impact on pregnancy outcome. Sleep Med. 2014;15(8):853–9.
4. Oyieng' o DO, Kirwa K, Tong I, Martin S, Rojas-Suarez JA, Bourjeily G. Restless legs symptoms and pregnancy and neonatal outcomes. Clin Ther. 2016;38(2):256–64.
5. Berle JO, Mykletun A, Daltveit AK, Rasmussen S, Holsten F, Dahl AA. Neonatal outcomes in offspring of women with anxiety and depression during pregnancy. A linkage study from The Nord-Trondelag Health Study (HUNT) and Medical Birth Registry of Norway. Arch Womens Ment Health. 2005;8(3):181–9. https://doi.org/10.1007/s00737-005-0090-z.
6. Ding XX, Wu YL, Xu SJ, et al. Maternal anxiety during pregnancy and adverse birth outcomes: a systematic review and meta-analysis of prospective cohort studies. J Affect Disord. 2014;159:103–10. https://doi.org/10.1016/j.jad.201.4.02.0.27.
7. Mcelhatton PR. Pregnancy: (2) general principles of drug use in pregnancy. Pharmaceutical J. 2003;270(7236):232.
8. Gidai J, Acs N, Banhidy F, Czeizel AE. No association found between the use of very large doses of diazepam by 112 pregnant women for a suicide attempt and congenital abnormalities in their offspring. Toxicol Ind Health. 2008;24:29–39.
9. Hartz SC, Heinonen OP, Shapiro S, Siskind JV, Slone D. Antenatal exposure to meprobamate and chlordiazepoxide in relation to malformations, mental development, and childhood mortality. N Engl J Med. 1975;292:726–8.
10. Brandlistuen RE, Ystrom E, Hernandez-Diaz S, Skurtveit S, Selmer R, Handal M, et al. Association of prenatal exposure to benzodiazepines and child internalizing problems: a sibling-controlled cohort study. PLoS One. 2017;12(7):e0181042. https://doi.org/10.1371/journal.pone.0181042.

11. The Organization of Teratology Information Specialists (OTIS) MotherToBaby. http://mothertobaby.org/fact-sheets/benzodiazepines-pregnancy/US. Department of Health and Human Services. Accessed 20 Aug 2018.
12. Vythilingum B. Anxiety disorders in pregnancy and the postnatal period. CME. 2009;27(10):450–2.
13. Pichetti DL, Hensley JG, Bainbridge JL, Lee KA, Manconi M, McGregor JA, et al. Consensus clinical practice guidelines for the diagnosis and treatment of restless legs syndrome/Willis Ekbom disease during pregnancy and lactation. Sleep Med Rev. 2015;22:64–7.
14. Gupta R, Dhyani M, Kendzerska T, Pandi-Perumal SR, BaHammam AS, Srivanitchapoom P, Pandey S, Hallett M. Restless legs syndrome and pregnancy: prevalence, possible pathophysiological mechanisms, and treatment. Act Neurol Scand. 2016;133:320–9. https://doi.org/10.1111/ane.12520.
15. Berger K, Luedemann J, Trenkwalder C, et al. Sex and the risk of restless legs syndrome in the general population. Arch Intern Med. 2004;164(2):196–202. https://doi.org/10.1001/archinte.164.2.196.
16. Sateia MJ. International classification of sleep disorders-third edition. Chest. 2015;146(5):1387–94.
17. Sikandrar R, Khealani BA, Wasay M. Predictors of restless legs syndrome in pregnancy: a hospital-based cross-sectional survey from Pakistan. Sleep Med. 2009;10(6):676–8.
18. Montplaisir J, Boucher S, Poirier G, Lavigne G, Lapierre O, Lesperance P. Clinical, polysomnographic, and genetic characteristics of restless legs syndrome: a study of 133 patients diagnosed with new standard criteria. Mov Disord. 1997;12(1):61–5.
19. Neau JP, Marion P, Mathis S, Julian A, Godeneche G, Larrieu D, Meurice JC, Paquereau J, Ingrand P. Restless legs syndrome, and pregnancy: follow-up of pregnant women before and after delivery. Eur Neurol. 2010;64:361–6. https://doi.org/10.1159/000322124.
20. Pantaleo NP, Hening WA, Allen RP, Early CJ. Pregnancy accounts for most of the gender differences in the prevalence of familial RLS. Sleep Med. 2010;11(3):310–3. https://doi.org/10.1016/j.sleep.2009.04.005.
21. Hubner A, Krafft A, Esther Werth SG, Zimmermann R, Bassetti C. Characteristics and determinants of restless legs syndrome in pregnancy. Neurology. 2013;80:738–42.
22. Grover A, Clark-Bilodeau C, D'Ambrosio CM. Restless leg syndrome in pregnancy. Obstet Med. 2015;8(3):121–5. https://doi.org/10.1177/1753495X15587452.
23. Manconi M, Ulfberg J, Berger K, Ghorayeb I, Wesström J, Fulda S, Allen RP, Pollmächer T. When gender matters: restless legs syndrome. Report of the "RLS and woman" workshop endorsed by the European RLS Study Group. Sleep Med Rev. 2012;16(4):297–307.
24. Pereira JC Jr, Rocha e Silva IR, Pradella-Hallinan M. Transient Willis–Ekbom's disease (restless legs syndrome) during pregnancy may be caused by estradiol-mediated dopamine overmodulation. Med Hypotheses. 2013;80(2):205–8.
25. Cesnik E, Casetta I, Turri M, Govoni V, Granieri E, Strambi LF, Manconi M. Transient RLS during pregnancy is a risk factor for the chronic idiopathic form. Neurology. 2010;75(23):2117.
26. Balendran J, Champion D, Jaaniste T, Welsh A. A common sleep disorder in pregnancy: restless legs syndrome and its predictors. Aust NZ J Obstet Gynaecol. 2011;51:262–4.
27. Suzuki K, Ohida T, Sone T, Takemura S, Yokoyama E, Miyake T, Harano S, Motojima S, Suga M, Ibuka E. The prevalence of restless legs syndrome among pregnant women in Japan and the relationship between restless legs syndrome and sleep problems. Sleep. 2003;26(6):673–7.
28. Uglane MT, Westad S, Backe B. Restless legs syndrome in pregnancy is a frequent disorder with a good prognosis. Acta Obstet Gynecol Scand. 2011;90:1046–8. https://doi.org/10.1111/j.1600-0412.2011.01157.x.
29. Manconi M, Govoni V, De Vito A, Economou NT, Cesnik E, Casetta I, Mollica G, Ferini-Strambi L, Granieri E. Restless legs syndrome and pregnancy. Neurology. 2004;63(6):1065–9. https://doi.org/10.1212/01.WNL.0000138427.83574.A6.
30. Becker JB. Direct effect of 17β-estradiol on striatum: sex differences in dopamine release. Synapse. 1990;5:157–64. https://doi.org/10.1002/syn.890050211.

31. Dzaja A, Wehrle R, Lancel M, Pollmächer T. Elevated Estradiol plasma levels in women with restless legs during pregnancy. Sleep. 2009;32(2):169–74.
32. Daubian-Nose' P, Frank MK, Maculano-Esteves A. Sleep disorders: a review of the interface between restless legs syndrome and iron metabolism. Sleep Sci. 2014;7:234–7. http://creativecommons.org/licenses/by-nc-nd/3.0/
33. Ozer I, Guzel I, Orhan G, Erkılınç S, Öztekin N, Ak F, Taşçı Y. A prospective case-control questionnaire study for restless leg syndrome on 600 pregnant women. J Matern Fetal Neonatal Med. 2016;30(24):2895–9. https://doi.org/10.3109/14767058.2016.1170801.
34. Çakmak B, Metin ZF, Karatafl A, Özsoy Z, Demirtürk F. Restless leg syndrome in pregnancy. Perinatal J. 2014;22(1):1–5. https://doi.org/10.2399/prn.14.0221001.
35. Mehmood T, Auerbach M, Earley CJ, Allen RP. Response to intravenous iron in patients with iron deficiency anemia (IDA) and restless leg syndrome (Willis–Ekbom disease). Sleep Med. 2014;15(12):1473–6. https://doi.org/10.1016/j.sleep.2014.08.012.
36. Grim K, Lee B, Sung AY, Kotagal S. Treatment of childhood-onset restless legs syndrome and periodic limb movement disorder using intravenous iron sucrose. Sleep Med. 2013;14(11):1100–4. https://doi.org/10.1016/j.sleep.2013.06.006.
37. Vadasz D, Ries V, Oertel WH. Intravenous iron sucrose for restless legs syndrome in pregnant women with low serum ferritin. Sleep Med. 2013;14(11):1214–6. https://doi.org/10.1016/j.sleep.2013.05.018.
38. Trenkwalder C, Paulus W. Restless legs syndrome: pathophysiology, clinical presentation, and management. Nat Rev Neurol. 2010;6:337–46.
39. Winkelmann J, Barbara Schormair B, Meitinger T. Genome-wide association study of restless legs syndrome identifies common variants in three genomic regions. Nat Genet. 2007;39:1000–6.
40. Schormair B, Kemlink D, Juliane Winkelmann J. PTPRD (protein tyrosine phosphatase receptor type delta) is associated with restless legs syndrome. Nat Genet. 2008;40:946–8.
41. Earley CJ, Silber MH. Restless legs syndrome: understanding its consequences and the need for better treatment. Sleep Med. 2010;11:807–15. https://doi.org/10.1016/j.sleep.2010.07.007.
42. Lee KA, Zaffke ME, Baratte-Beebe K. Restless legs syndrome and sleep disturbance in pregnancy. J Womens Health Gend Based Med. 2001;10(4):335–41.
43. Minár M, Habánová H, Rusňák I, Planck K, Peter Valkovič P. Prevalence and impact of restless legs syndrome in pregnancy. Neuroendocrinol Lett. 2013;34(5):366–71.
44. Liu G, Li L, Zhang J, Xue R, Zhao X, Zhu K, Wang Y, Xiao L, Shangguan J. Restless legs syndrome and pregnancy or delivery complications in China: a representative survey. Sleep Med. 2016;17:158–62.
45. Neau JP, Porcheron A, Mathis S, Julian A, Meurice JC, Paquereau J, Godeneche G, Ciron J, Bouche G. Restless legs syndrome and pregnancy: a questionnaire study in the Poitiers District, France. Eur Neurol. 2010;64:268–74.
46. Nodine PM, Matthews EE. Common sleep disorders: management strategies and pregnancy outcomes. J Midwifery Womens Health. 2013;58:368–77.
47. Tan M, Bourjeily G. Shaking up perspectives on restless legs syndrome in pregnancy: commentary on Dunietz et al Restless legs syndrome and sleep-wake disturbances in pregnancy. J Clin Sleep Med. 2017;13(7):857–8.
48. Aukerman MM, Aukerman D, Bayard M, Tudiver F, Thorp I, Bailey B. Exercise and restless legs syndrome: a randomized controlled trial. J Am Board Fam Med. 2006f;19:487–93.
49. Western Australian Department of Health. Perinatal and infant mental health model of care – a framework. Perth: North Metropolitan Health Service, Western Australian Department of Health, Western Australia; 2016.
50. Snellen M, Thompson G, Murdoch N. The process of obtaining informed consent when prescribing psychopharmacology in pregnancy. In: Galbally M, et al., editors. Psychopharmacology and pregnancy. Berlin: Springer-Verlag; 2014. https://doi.org/10.1007/978-3-642-54562-7_7.
51. Taylor D, Paton C, Kapur S. Maudsley prescribing guidelines in psychiatry. 12th ed. Oxford UK: Wiley Blackwell; 2015.

52. Garcia Borreguero D, Ferini-Stranbi L, Kohnen R, O'Keefe S, Trenkwaider C, Hogyl B, et al. European guidelines on management of restless legs syndrome: report of a joint task force by the European Federation of Neurological Societies, the European Neurological Society and the European Sleep Research Society. Eur J Neurol. 2012;19:1385–96.
53. Saxen I, Saxen L. Association between maternal intake of diazepam and oral clefts. Lancet. 1975;2:498.
54. Lin AE, Peller AJ, Westgate MN, Houde K, Franz A, Holmes LB. Clonazepam use in pregnancy and the risk of malformations. Birth Defects Res A Clin Mol Teratol. 2004;70:534–6.
55. Freeman MP, Goez-Mogolion L, McInerney KA, Davies AC, Church TR, Sosinsky AZ, et al. Obstetrical and neonatal outcomes after benzodiazepine exposure during pregnancy: results from a prospective registry of women with psychiatric disorders. Gen Hosp Psychiatry. 2018;53:73–9.
56. Kallen B, Reis M. Neonatal complications after maternal concomitant use of SSRI and other central nervous system active drugs during the second or third trimester of pregnancy. J Clin Psychopharmacol. 2012;32(5):608–14. https://doi.org/10.1097/JCP.Ob013e3182668568.
57. Kallen B, Borg N, Reis M. The use of central nervous system active drugs during pregnancy. Pharmaceuticals. 2013;6(10):1221–86. https://doi.org/10.3390/ph6101221.
58. Calderon-Margalit R, Qui C, Ornoy A, Siscovick DS, Williams MA. Risk of preterm delivery and other adverse perinatal outcomes in relation to maternal use of psychotropic medication during pregnancy. Am J Obstet Gynecol. 2009;201(6):579.e1–8. https://doi.org/10.1016/j.ajpg.2009.06.061.
59. Iqbal MM, Tanveer Sobhamn T, Ryals T. Effects of commonly used benzodiazepines on the fetus, neonate and the nursing infant. Psychiatr Serv. 2002;53:39–49.
60. Birnbaum CS, Cohen LS, Bailey JW, Grush MD, Robertson LM, Stowe ZN. Serum concentrations of antidepressants and benzodiazepines in nursing infants: a case series. Pediatrics. 1999;104:e11. PMID: 10390297
61. Dostal M, Weber-Schoendorfer C, Sobesky J, Schaefer C. Pregnancy outcome following use of levodopa, pramipexole, ropinirole, and rotigotine for restless legs syndrome during pregnancy: a case series. Eur J Neurol. 2013;20:1241–6.
62. Allen RP, Earley C. Augmentation of the restless legs syndrome with Carbidopa/levodopa. Sleep. 1996;19(3):205.
63. Silver N, Allen RP, Senerth J, Earley CJ. A 10-year, longitudinal assessment of dopamine agonists and methadone in the treatment of restless legs syndrome. Sleep Med. 2011;12:440–4.
64. Walters AS, Winkelmann J, Trenkwalder C, Fry JM, Kataria V, Wagner M, et al. Long-term follow-up on restless legs syndrome patients treated with opioids. Mov Disord. 2001;16:1105–9.
65. Yang C, White DP, Winkelman JW. Antidepressants and periodic leg movements of sleep. Biol Psychiatry. 2005;58:510–4.

Suggested Reading

Pichetti DL, Hensley JG, Bainbridge JL, Lee KA, Manconi M, McGregor JA, et al. Consensus clinical practice guidelines for the diagnosis and treatment of restless legs syndrome/Willis Ekbom disease during pregnancy and lactation. Sleep Med Rev. 2015;22:64–7.

Part IV

Sleep Issues in Children and Adolescents

Insufficient Sleep in Adolescence: Individual Interventions and Interventions That Scale

9

Stephen Talsness and Conrad Iber

Clinical History

A 17-year-old male high school student with a history of depression, anxiety, and attention-deficit/hyperactivity disorder (ADHD) presented to the sleep clinic with his mother for concern of difficulty waking up in the morning. His parents had the most concern about his symptoms as he is unable to wake up by alarm, and his parents go to great lengths each morning to get him out of bed. Highlighting this concern, his mother states, "I am not sure he could function independently if we do not wake him up." Even when they awake him, there are mornings when he will appear to be awake and have full conversations with his parents before falling back asleep. He is unable to recall these conversations when asked about them later in the morning. He describes difficulty getting into bed before midnight and uses his cell phone in the first few hours after he gets in bed.

His mother notes that he has been a night person since about middle school. During that time, he began to have difficulty in school and to exhibit symptoms of depression and anxiety that were treated with psychotherapy and sertraline. About 6 months before the presentation, the antidepressant was discontinued, and he was diagnosed with ADHD and started on an amphetamine-dextroamphetamine salt. His symptoms of inattention were noted to have initiated during middle school as well. The stimulant was partially effective in addressing his difficulties with attention, yet his symptoms did not entirely remit despite the addition of guanfacine. There was a hesitancy to advance the dose of the stimulant, for fear of exacerbating his sleep difficulties.

S. Talsness (✉)
Department of Psychiatry, Minneapolis VA Health Care System, Minneapolis, MN, USA
e-mail: Stephen.Talsness@va.gov

C. Iber
Department of Medicine, M Health Fairview, Minneapolis, MN, USA

© Springer Nature Switzerland AG 2021
I. S. Khawaja, T. D. Hurwitz (eds.), *Sleep Disorders in Selected Psychiatric Settings*, https://doi.org/10.1007/978-3-030-59309-4_9

He started tracking his sleep with a smartwatch app that recorded variations in total sleep time of 6–8.5 hours over the past 2 weeks. He gets into bed around midnight during the week, spending time on his phone in bed and falling asleep at 1 am or later. He does not use sleep aids. He sleeps through the night and stays sleeping in bed despite repeated attempts by his parents at waking him. He ultimately gets out of bed around 7 am and drives to school for his first class at 7:50 am. He will frequently fall asleep in morning classes. He otherwise does not nap or doze off during the day. Epworth Sleepiness Scale score is 6 of 24. On weekends, he frequently stays up until 2 am or later, waking at noon or later without an alarm.

He denied symptoms suggestive of sleep-disordered breathing, nighttime sleep disruption, or cataplexy. Other than the weekday morning somniloquy, he denied a history of parasomnia. His medical history was unremarkable. His psychiatric history was devoid of hospitalization, a suicide attempt, or self-injury.

He is currently a junior in high school. He played hockey, yet stopped about 2 years ago because late-night practices got in the way of completing homework. He consumes between one and three caffeinated beverages per day, including colas in the evening. He denied tobacco, alcohol, and illicit drug use. Family history was positive for a delayed sleep phase preference in his father, yet he was negative for sleep-disordered breathing, narcolepsy, or restless leg syndrome.

Examination

The patient was generally well-appearing and in no distress. His body mass index was 21.5 kg/m^2, and the upper airway exam revealed a Mallampati class I airway, tonsils of grade 0–1, and normal nasal turbinates, septum, and airflow. Neck circumference was 35 cm. The mood was described as "good" and his affect pleasant and congruent. His cardiovascular, respiratory, abdominal, and neurologic exams were within the normal limits.

Questions

What three interventions might be useful in promoting sufficient sleep?
Which of his signs and symptoms might be ascribed to a sleep problem?
What risks would his sleep problem pose?

Diagnosis

The patient's symptoms and sleep schedule support a diagnosis of insufficient sleep and circadian misalignment with weekend sleep, suggesting delayed sleep-wake phase disorder (DSWPD). Normal adolescent sleep phase delay is compounded by early school start time, which amputates natural morning sleep time and is aggravated by evening screen exposure and caffeine, resulting in as little as 6 hours of sleep on weekdays as compared to the recommended sleep duration of 8–10 hours in this age group [1].This would result in a 10-hour sleep debt over 1 week. Although the duration of sleep is increased on weekends, his unrestricted waking time uncovers a tendency for sleep phase delay. Insufficient sleep and weekend delay in sleep offset in high school students have been associated with mood disturbances and impaired performance [2], and reduction in depressive symptoms has been reported when student are offered more sleep opportunity by delaying school schedules [3]. In this case, the student experiences sleep as a restorative when waking on weekend mornings with two additional hours of sleep. The additional sleep is associated with the elimination of episodes of somniloquy likely due to the impact of increased sleep duration in preventing confusional arousals from sleep. The onset of mood disturbances and attention difficulties later in adolescence with an absence of symptoms in early childhood suggests a role of insufficient sleep and circadian misalignment in the genesis of these issues.

Remarks

A normal developmental sleep phase delay of 1–2 hours in adolescents has been noted across cultures and settings and long before the presence of mobile electronic equipment in the bedroom. Circadian misaligned social activities, including early school start time, curtail restorative activities and impair cognition and mood. The effect is more pronounced in rural communities, where prolonged bus transit time can further limit sleep opportunity. This can be exacerbated further by commonly used evening electronic equipment, poorly timed evening caffeine use, and extracurricular activities and sports that hold morning practices during the week. Concerning caffeine use patterns in adolescents is highly prevalent with typical use not occurring until evening [4].The summation of these biological, psychosocial, and societal pressures results in insufficient sleep during the week with weekends commonly consisting of a delayed sleep phase, giving rise to social jet lag, and an increased duration of sleep, as a function of sleep debt, accumulated during the week (see Fig. 9.1).

Insufficient sleep in this setting has been associated with sleepiness, mood disturbances, and inattention, all evident in this case, yet also academic and behavioral problems, substance use, motor vehicle accidents, overweight, and immune system dysfunction. In a large survey of over 27,000 adolescents [5], insufficient sleep was found to increase the risk of substance abuse and hopelessness. It was also associated with a greater than a fivefold increased risk of suicide attempts. The use of bright screens before bedtime can aggravate sleep phase delay through increased evening alertness and delays in sleep onset. A longitudinal study of over 2800 adolescents found an association between screen time and insomnia symptoms, short sleep duration, and depressive symptoms [6].

Individual recommendations around behavior change to improve sleep hygiene and correct insufficient sleep, coupled with modifications of the circadian phase, can be effective. Evening melatonin administered at a low dose has been shown to

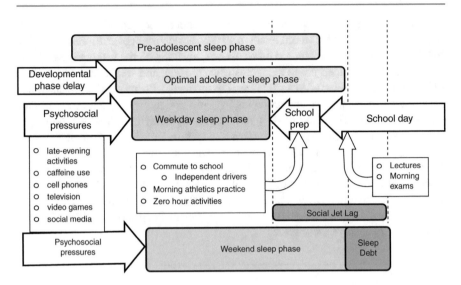

Fig. 9.1 Social jet lag: the shift work of adolescence. Myriad psychosocial pressures exacerbate a biological circadian phase delay during adolescence. Early school start times and morning activities before school serve to amputate the total sleep duration during the week. Catching up on sleep on weekends results in a social jet lag, and total sleep time is often increased on weekends, reflecting a sleep debt built up from insufficient sleep over the school week

advance the dim light melatonin onset. Morning light exposure has also been experimentally validated. However, a review of the literature and meta-analysis of these approaches was conducted, and current clinical practice guidelines are weak in their recommendation for these treatments [7]. Moreover, the durability of these therapies has not been thoroughly assessed. In a study of bright light therapy coupled with cognitive behavioral therapy for insomnia, the adolescent participants with DSWPD were followed for 6 months, and while the treatment was effective, 13% receiving treatment still met criteria for DSPWD, and attrition at 6-month follow-up was a concern [8]. As has been understood from clinical experience for some time [9], light therapy can be effective, yet "once bedtime reaches an acceptable hour, rigid adherence to a schedule remains mandatory." With the dynamic nature of adolescent development, adherence to severe behavioral changes is understandably problematic.

Another approach is to view the problem as a social determinant of health, affecting not only the patient described in this case but the entire population of 15 million high school students in the United States, 89% of which are estimated to have an insufficient sleep. Delaying school start times has been shown to address this concern resulting in about 21 minutes longer sleep for every hour the start time is delayed [10]. A review of eight observational studies found an association between delayed school start times and greater psychological health [11]. Another review of the literature found that later start times were associated with "improved attendance, less tardiness, less falling asleep in class, better grades, and fewer motor vehicle crashes" [12]. Unfortunately, while the American Academy of Pediatrics recommends that teenagers not start their school day before 8:30 am, only 17.7% of schools comply [13]. Delay in school start time for middle and high school offers a substantial population strategy to improve adolescent health and well-being [14]. This presents an opportunity for sleep physicians and psychiatrists to engage with local school districts around school start times and the timing of other activities and with adolescents and their parents on education related to sleep and circadian biology.

Pearls
- Normal biological changes in adolescence give rise to a sleep phase delay of about 1–2 hours.
- Evening light exposure delays the circadian sleep phase.
- Screen use is also correlated with short sleep duration, insomnia, and depressive symptoms.
- Insufficient sleep is associated with a greater than fivefold risk of suicide attempts.
- Morning light therapy and evening melatonin can advance the sleep phase.
- Adolescent sleep increases by about 21 minutes for each hour the school start time is delayed.
- Later school start times are associated with greater psychological health, better grades, and fewer motor vehicle accidents.

References

1. Paruthi S, Brooks LJ, D'Ambrosio C, et al. Consensus statement of the American Academy of sleep medicine on the recommended amount of sleep for healthy children: methodology and discussion. J Clin Sleep Med. 2016;12(11):1549–61. https://doi.org/10.5664/jcsm.6288.
2. O'Brien EM, Mindell JA. Sleep and risk-taking behavior in adolescents. Behav Sleep Med. 2005;3(3):113–33. https://doi.org/10.1207/s15402010bsm0303_1.
3. Wahlstrom KL, Berger AT, Widome R. Relationships between school start time, sleep duration, and adolescent behaviors. Sleep Heal. 2017;3(3):216–21. https://doi.org/10.1016/j.sleh.2017.03.002.
4. Bryant Ludden A, Wolfson AR. Understanding adolescent caffeine use: connecting use patterns with expectancies, reasons, and sleep. Heal Educ Behav. 2010;37(3):330–42. https://doi.org/10.1177/1090198109341783.
5. Winsler A, Deutsch A, Vorona RD, Payne PA, Szklo-Coxe M. Sleepless in Fairfax: the difference one more hour of sleep can make for teen hopelessness, suicidal ideation, and substance use. J Youth Adolesc. 2014;44(2):362–78. https://doi.org/10.1007/s10964-014-0170-3.
6. Li X, Buxton OM, Lee S, Chang AM, Berger LM, Hale L. Sleep mediates the association between adolescent screen time and depressive symptoms. Sleep Med. 2019;57:51–60. https://doi.org/10.1016/j.sleep.2019.01.029.
7. Auger RR, Burgess HJ, Emens JS, Deriy LV, Thomas SM, Sharkey KM. Clinical practice guideline for the treatment of intrinsic circadian rhythm sleep-wake disorders: advanced sleep-wake phase disorder (ASWPD), Delayed Sleep-Wake Phase Disorder (DSWPD), Non-24-Hour Sleep-Wake Rhythm Disorder (N24SWD), and irregular sleep-W. J Clin Sleep Med. 2015;11(10):1199–236. https://doi.org/10.5664/jcsm.5100.

8. Gradisar M, Dohnt H, Gardner G, et al. A randomized controlled trial of cognitive-behavior therapy plus bright light therapy for adolescent delayed sleep phase disorder. Sleep. 2011;34(12):1671–80. https://doi.org/10.5665/sleep.1432.

9. Hauri PJ. Delayed and advanced sleep phase syndromes. In: Sleep Disorders: Upjohn; 1992. Kalamazoo, Michigan.

10. Nahmod NG, Lee S, Master L, Chang AM, Hale L, Buxton OM. Later high school start times associated with longer actigraphic sleep duration in adolescents. Sleep. 2019;42(2):1–10. https://doi.org/10.1093/sleep/zsy212.

11. Berger AT, Widome R, Troxel WM. School start time and psychological health in adolescents. Curr Sleep Med Rep. 2018;4(2):110–7. https://doi.org/10.1007/s40675-018-0115-6.

12. Wheaton AG, Chapman DP, Croft JB, Chief B, Branch S. School start times, sleep, behavioral, health, and academic outcomes: a review of the literature. J Sch Health. 2016;86(5):363–81. https://doi.org/10.1111/josh.12388.

13. Wheaton AG, Ferro GA, Croft JB. School start times for middle school and high school students – the United States, 2011–12 school year. MMWR Morb Mortal Wkly Rep. 2015;64(30):809–13. PMCID: PMC5779581

14. Berger AT, Widome R, Troxel WM. Delayed school start times and adolescent health. In: Sleep and health: Elsevier; 2019. p. 447–54. https://doi.org/10.1016/B978-0-12-815373-4.00033-2.

What Is Wrong with My Child? Narcolepsy and Its Emotional Burden on Parents

10

Anna Wani, Rachel Rosen, and S. Kamal Naqvi

Chapter Outline

Understand the diagnostic and treatment challenges of pediatric narcolepsy with a specific emphasis on the emotional burden of parents.

Clinical History

A 12-year-old female has been followed in the sleep disorders clinic since age 6 for excessive daytime sleepiness and poor school performance. Significant daytime sleepiness was first identified when the child started kindergarten, as she would frequently sleep in class, despite the adequate duration of nocturnal sleep. She was initially evaluated by an Ear, Nose, and Throat (ENT) specialist for symptoms of daytime sleepiness, mouth breathing, and tonsillar and adenoidal hypertrophy. A polysomnogram (PSG) was completed at an outside facility revealing no evidence of sleep apnea. The child then underwent adenotonsillectomy.

A second polysomnogram followed by a multiple sleep latency test (MSLT) was completed as daytime sleepiness did not improve with surgery. The child presented to the sleep disorders center for abnormal MSLT findings from the outside facility.

A. Wani
UT Southwestern Medical Center/Children's Health, Sleep Disorders Center, Dallas, TX, USA

R. Rosen
Children's Health, Sleep Disorder Center, Dallas, TX, USA

S. K. Naqvi (✉)
Department of Pediatrics, UT Southwestern Medical Center/Children's Health, Sleep Disorders Center, Dallas, TX, USA
e-mail: kamal.naqvi@utsouthwestern.edu

© Springer Nature Switzerland AG 2021
I. S. Khawaja, T. D. Hurwitz (eds.), *Sleep Disorders in Selected Psychiatric Settings*, https://doi.org/10.1007/978-3-030-59309-4_10

A repeat PSG/MSLT was completed at the pediatric sleep center, given the child's young age at initial testing. The mother denied previous head injury, influenza, or Pandemrix.

The child has had a progression of symptoms over time to include excessive daytime sleepiness, fragmented nocturnal sleep, sleep paralysis, and cataplexy. Cataplexy includes head and jaw-dropping with laughter. The child will blunt her emotions to avoid the laughter and subsequent cataleptic event.

Routine follow-up at the tertiary center has been difficult as the family lives far in the rural part of the state. In addition, there are complex social stressors, including the incarceration of a close household family member due to drug offenses. Mother is concerned that the child is sad and anxious due to lifelong diagnosis and changes in the family dynamic. The child reports an imaginary family as a coping mechanism.

Diagnostic Testing Performed

Polysomnogram
    Multiple sleep latency test
    Narcolepsy HLA DNA panel
    MRI brain
    Electroencephalography (EEG)
    Actigraphy

Results

PSG (at diagnosis) (Fig. 10.1). No evidence of sleep-disordered breathing. Sleep architecture and stage distribution were normal. REM sleep latency was slightly short at 71 minutes. No periodic limb movements were seen.

MSLT (at diagnosis) (Fig. 10.2). The patient was given five nap opportunities. She fell asleep in all naps and had REM sleep in all five naps. The average latency to sleep is 0 minutes, and REM sleep latency is 1 minute.

Narcolepsy HLA DNA PCR – POSITIVE for HLA-DQB1*06:02.

MRI brain without contrast revealed no significant intracranial abnormalities.

Epilepsy monitoring unit admission. The patient had several clinical events characterized by a loss of tone and slumping over to the bed when she was emotionally excited. Clowns coming into her room triggered this. After interacting with the clowns for several seconds, the patient is seen losing the tone of her upper body following laughter. No ictal EEG changes were seen during the events.

Actigraphy revealed inconsistent sleep/wake patterns.

Narcolepsy Type 1

Narcolepsy is considered a rare condition, but it is not as uncommon as one might think [1, 2]. About 1 in 2000 people in the United States is estimated to have narcolepsy [3].

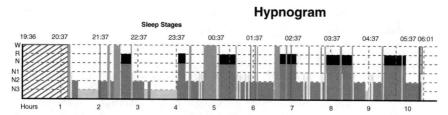

Fig. 10.1 Repeat PSG

SLEEP ARCHITECTURE

Sleep Summary			
Light Out	8:48PM	Ligts On	6:00AM
Total Study Time	552 mins	Time in Bed	626 mins
Total Sleep Time	479 mins	Sleep Effciency	86.7%
Total Wake Time	73 mins	Sleep Latency	04 mins
		REM Latency	57 mins

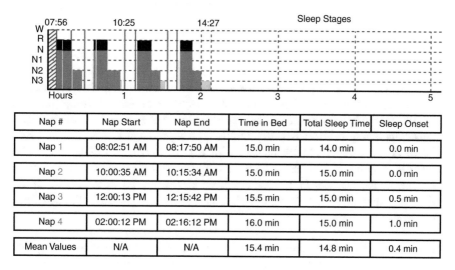

Nap #	Nap Start	Nap End	Time in Bed	Total Sleep Time	Sleep Onset
Nap 1	08:02:51 AM	08:17:50 AM	15.0 min	14.0 min	0.0 min
Nap 2	10:00:35 AM	10:15:34 AM	15.0 min	15.0 min	0.0 min
Nap 3	12:00:13 PM	12:15:42 PM	15.5 min	15.0 min	0.5 min
Nap 4	02:00:12 PM	02:16:12 PM	16.0 min	15.0 min	1.0 min
Mean Values	N/A	N/A	15.4 min	14.8 min	0.4 min

Fig. 10.2 Repeat MSLT

Narcolepsy is a lifelong disorder that is underdiagnosed and misunderstood. It can take months to years before a proper diagnosis can be made for those affected. There is a heavy burden placed on children who are diagnosed with narcolepsy, which extends to their parents [4].

Sometimes, narcolepsy presents after acute illness and is characterized by sudden weight gain and persistent sleepiness. It may or may not be associated with cataplexy initially (Table 10.1).

Table 10.1 Diagnostic criteria: Narcolepsy type 1

The patient has daily periods of irrepressible need to sleep or daytime lapses into sleep occurring for at least 3 months
The presence of one or both of the following:
The cataplexy and a mean sleep latency of 8 minutes or less and two or more sleep-onset rapid eye movement periods (SOREMPs) on a multiple sleep latency test (MSLT)
A SOREMP (within 15 min of sleep onset) on the preceding nocturnal polysomnogram (PSG) may replace one of the SOREMPs on the MSLT
Cerebrospinal fluid (CSF) hypocretin-1 concentration, measured by immunoreactivity, is either 110 pg/mL or less or less than one-third of mean values obtained in healthy subjects with the same standardized assay[1]

Table 10.2 Differential diagnosis

Inadequate sleep
Idiopathic hypersomnia
Obstructive sleep apnea
Depression or other psychiatric disorders
Attention deficit hyperactivity disorder
Learning disorder
Epilepsy
Chronic fatigue syndrome

Discussion

When parents bring their children for evaluation of narcolepsy, they are usually exasperated, as narcolepsy has significant impacts on a child's daytime function, including school performance and behavior. Typically, they have been to other specialists, including neurologists, psychiatrists, or psychologists, who may not specialize in the disorder. Many present with a prior diagnosis (Table 10.2). The diagnosis may not be addressing all the issues their child is having, and the family is desperate for answers. In the case described above, the child was first diagnosed with sleep-disordered breathing, and despite undergoing adenotonsillectomy, she was persistently sleepy.

Testing for narcolepsy is lengthy. The overnight sleep study and multiple sleep latency tests require the parent to remain present all night and the following day. Household responsibilities, including the care of other children, must be delegated. Multiple sleep latency testing can be taxing on parents as the child is asked to stay awake and sleep only on cue. When the repeat PSG/MSLT was completed on the child described in the case, she was irritable and physically belligerent with the parent when asked not to sleep between scheduled naps.

The emotional toll continues with the diagnosis. The label of narcolepsy is a permanent one. It is distressing for any parent to have a child diagnosed with a chronic illness. Treatment of narcolepsy can be burdensome and heavily dependent on buy-in from parents and educators. Individual plans involve educating all family members, teachers, coaches, and friends, as well as behavioral and medication treatment. The standard treatment for narcolepsy with cataplexy is sodium oxybate. This medication requires twice-nightly administration, in which the parent will wake up in the middle of sleep to give a second dose. In the case described above, the patient would likely benefit from sodium oxybate therapy, but it is not recommended given the high-risk family situation, including past drug offenses.

Finally, the functional decline in the child can be quite worrisome for the parent watch. Children may have a significant drop in their academic performance. Additionally, comorbid psychiatric conditions can place added stress on the family unit. In the case described, the baseline family situation is already complicated and stressful. A child with a chronic illness that has a specific impact on the already truncated family structure is significantly burdensome. In addition to routine follow-up for the child's progress and well-being, it is crucial to address caregiver fatigue and the emotional burden placed on parents whose children carry the diagnosis of narcolepsy.

Pearls
- Timing: The family seeks multiple specialist opinions before finally reaching a pediatric sleep center. In many small cities, a sleep specialist does not even exist. It takes months to several years before a correct diagnosis reached.
- School: Symptoms of narcolepsy may be mistaken as laziness or a learning disability. School staff presumes poor parenting, inadequate sleep hygiene, and lack of discipline at home that leads to parental guilt and anxiety. Declining performance despite the child making a reasonable effort adds to parental frustration and stress.
- Diagnosis: Sleep study, including nocturnal testing and daytime nap study, can be very cumbersome for a parent.
- Treatment: The FDA does not approve some very effective medications for pediatric patients. Although understanding the family situation is vital in chronic illness, it is especially crucial in narcolepsy because stimulants and sodium oxybate require a stable home environment where parents can take responsibility for safeguarding and dosing the medication.
- Cataplexy: Cataplexy can lead to embarrassment and become a constant fear for the patient and the parent during various social situations. Parents are often concerned about cataplexy and safety during sports activities. Additionally, a child may hold back emotions, including laughter, as discussed in the case, which can be distressing for a parent to witness.

- Independence: Parents feel obligated to supervise a child with narcolepsy even into adult age, which limits a young adult's autonomy. Parents are involved in supervising medications, college or work performance, and social interaction. Driving-safety is a significant concern and source of stress and anxiety for the parent.
- Psychological well-being: Patients with narcolepsy may have low self-esteem and frequently are depressed, which is challenging for parents.
- Obesity: Obesity is a common comorbid condition in the setting of narcolepsy, which can lead to other chronic conditions such as diabetes and hypertension, further complicating the clinical picture.

References

1. American Academy of Sleep Medicine. International classification of sleep disorders. 3rd ed. Darien: American Academy of Sleep Medicine; 2014.
2. Sheldon S, Kryger M, Ferber R, Gozal D. Principles and practice of pediatric sleep medicine. 2nd ed. Philadelphia: Saunders; 2014.
3. Jaquez S, Thakre T, Krishna J. Sleep disorders in adolescents. Cham: Springer; 2017. Chapter 2
4. Plazzi G, et al. Clinical characteristics and burden of illness in pediatric patients with narcolepsy. Pediatr Neurol. 85:21–32. https://doi.org/10.1016/j.pediatrneurol.2018.06.008.

Part V

Medication Induced Sleep Problems

Stimulant-Induced Sleep Disorder in Children with ADHD

Natasha Thrower, Edore Onigu-Otite, Michelle Nazario, Sophia Banu, and Asim A. Shah

Introduction

Sleep plays an essential part in optimal childhood development including in children with ADHD. A number of systematic reviews have demonstrated that children with ADHD report more sleep problems than children without ADHD, with the most common complaint being delayed sleep onset [1, 2]. As many as 70% of children with ADHD experience sleep difficulties [3, 4], making sleep problems the most common among the conditions associated with ADHD [5–8]. Systematic reviews indicate that children with ADHD have significantly higher bedtime

N. Thrower
Pediatric and Adolescent Health Center, Pasadena, TX, USA

Menninger Department of Psychiatry & Behavioral Sciences - Baylor College of Medicine, Houston, TX, USA

E. Onigu-Otite
Menninger Department of Psychiatry & Behavioral Sciences - Baylor College of Medicine, Houston, TX, USA

Ben Taub Neuropsychiatry Center, Houston, TX, USA

M. Nazario
Menninger Department of Psychiatry & Behavioral Sciences - Baylor College of Medicine, Houston, TX, USA

Ben Taub General Hospital, Houston, TX, USA

S. Banu
Menninger Department of Psychiatry & Behavioral Sciences, Baylor College of Medicine, Ben Taub Hospital Center, Department of Psychiatry, Houston, TX, USA

A. A. Shah (✉)
Menninger Department of Psychiatry & Behavioral Sciences, Baylor College of Medicine, Houston, TX, USA
e-mail: aashah@bcm.edu

© Springer Nature Switzerland AG 2021
I. S. Khawaja, T. D. Hurwitz (eds.), *Sleep Disorders in Selected Psychiatric Settings*, https://doi.org/10.1007/978-3-030-59309-4_11

resistance, more sleep onset difficulties, difficulties with morning awakenings, sleep disordered breathing, and daytime sleepiness compared with the controls [9]. Children with ADHD also have significantly lower sleep efficiency on polysomnography, actual sleep time on actigraphy, and average times to fall asleep for the Multiple Sleep Latency Test than the controls [10].

While insomnia is a well-known side effect of psychostimulants, 28% of medication-free ADHD patients suffer from sleep difficulties as well [9]. Children with ADHD may find it more difficult than typically developing children to slow their thoughts and to settle for sleep at bedtime. Furthermore, sleep disorders and psychiatric conditions which may impact sleep are more common in children with ADHD. When evaluating sleep issues in children who are treated for ADHD with stimulant medications, it is important to consider alternative etiologies and to screen for comorbid conditions. A failure to accurately diagnosis and treat a preexisting or co-occurring sleep problem may exacerbate ADHD symptoms, and compromise ADHD treatment efficacy, leading to greater functional impairment [11]. Generating accurate differential diagnoses is an essential step in evaluating sleep problems in children with ADHD [12].

The Case of a 9-Year-Old Boy with ADHD

History

A 9-year-old boy with attention-deficit/hyperactivity disorder (ADHD), combined presentation, and oppositional defiant disorder presents with a complaint of marked insomnia. Two months ago, after starting 36 mg of methylphenidate ER (Concerta®), his parents observed a 2-hour delay in sleep onset each night. Behavioral interventions such as scheduling bedtime, limiting screen-time, and caffeine intake did not sufficiently address the patient's insomnia. The patient was diagnosed with mild obstructive sleep apnea last year and underwent an adenotonsillectomy which improved his snoring and quality of sleep until recently. His parents say they are reluctant to try another stimulant medication because their son's ADHD symptoms have dramatically improved on Concerta. The child's parents would like to know what can be done to address his sleep issues.

Mental Status Examination

- Appearance: appears stated age, casually dressed in age-appropriate clothing
- Orientation: alert and oriented to person, location, and date
- Social relatedness: limited engagement, adequate cooperation with the interview, good eye contact
- Motor: gait grossly normal, no abnormal movements noted
- Activity: seated upright in chair, with frequent fidgeting of hands and feet
- Speech: normal volume, rate, and tone

- Mood: irritable ("annoyed with mom")
- Affect: angry
- Thought processes: concrete, goal-directed (stays on topic in an age/developmentally appropriate manner)
- Thought content: denies any suicidal content, intent, or plan. Denies any homicidal ideation. No delusions elicited
- Perceptual disturbance: denies any auditory or visual hallucinations. Denies paranoia
- Estimate of intellectual functioning: average
- Insight: limited
- Judgment: appropriate for age and developmental level

Tests and Results

Polysomnography

Nocturnal Session Sleep Characteristics

The patient was put to bed, and the lights were turned off at 21:28 hours. After 98.0 minutes the patient fell asleep achieving a period of non-REM (NREM) sleep. The total sleep time was 5.03 hours accounting for 58.8% of the monitoring time (expected values greater than 90%). Both REM and NREM sleep characteristics were recorded. The sleep stage distribution was atypical for age with 13.1% stage REM sleep recorded (expected range 18–25%). During the study, there were 12.9 arousals per hour of sleep (significant values greater than 14 per hour of sleep). Sleep-disordered breathing was associated with 2.2 arousals per hour of sleep. Periodic limb movements were associated with 0.2 arousals per hour of sleep.

Respiratory Analysis The patient was recorded while sleeping on the back and sides. Snoring was recorded. During wakefulness, the respiratory rate was 22 breaths per minute. During sleep, the respiratory rate was 16–20 breaths per minute. The baseline oxygen saturation was 97%. The oxygen nadir was 94%. The patient spent 0% of the total sleep time with oxygen saturation values of less than 90%. The transcutaneous pCO_2 values were elevated to as high as 46 mmHg. During 0% of the monitoring time, pCO_2 values were elevated above 50 mmHg (significant values >25%). During sleep, no obstructive apneas, mixed apneas, or central apneas were recorded. Fifteen obstructive hypopneas were recorded. The apnea hypopnea index was 2.98. The obstructive apnea-hypopnea index was 2.98. The respiratory disturbance index was 2.98 (2.98 obstructive respiratory events per hour of sleep). Respiratory events were recorded more frequently in the supine position (5.52 obstructive events per hour).

Cardiac Analysis The heart rate was typically in the range of 65–82 beats per minute. No significant cardiac arrhythmias were recorded.

Limb Movement Analysis During sleep, there were 19 periodic limb movements recorded (3.7 per hour of sleep; significant values greater than 5.0 per hour of sleep).

EEG Recordings The occipital dominant rhythm was 10 Hz. There were no focal or lateralizing features. No epileptiform abnormalities were recorded.

Impression During sleep, mild obstructive sleep apnea (2.98 obstructive events per hour of sleep and snoring) was recorded. The minimum oxygen value was 94%; pCO_2 values were not significantly elevated. There was no central sleep apnea. No cardiac arrhythmias were recorded. The EEG findings were normal. There was no significant occurrence of periodic limb movements during sleep.

Recommendations
1. Evaluation of the upper airway
2. If the patient undergoes surgery, consider follow up study in 6–8 weeks
3. Other options: trial of Continuous positive airway pressure/Bilevel positive airway pressure

---

Clinical Question and Case Discussion

How can clinicians appropriately assess and address stimulant-induced insomnia in children with ADHD?

As a first step, the patient's record was reviewed and additional historical information obtained to assess the cause of the sleep difficulty. However, no other psychiatric, medical, environmental, or behavioral factors which could explain the abrupt sleep disturbance were identified. The parents were re-educated regarding the potential risks of stimulant treatment and the impact of poor sleep on cognition and behavior, but they were reluctant to change the medication or adjust the dose when presented with these options. The patient's parents agreed with the plan to administer Concerta on school days (Monday to Friday) and to track the child's sleep patterns using a sleep diary. The sleep diary findings illustrated a pattern of significant sleep onset delay associated with days in which the medication was taken as compared to weekends when it was not. Melatonin 1–3 mg for methylphenidate-induced insomnia was subsequently prescribed to which the patient and parents reported good tolerability and effect.

Discussion

Problematic sleep itself can result in deficits of executive function, cognition, and behavioral regulations which are also characteristic of ADHD. A baseline sleep assessment should be performed during the initial ADHD evaluation, before the initiation of treatment with stimulant medications, in order to identify underlying sleep pathology which might be responsible for causing ADHD-like symptoms and improve symptoms with treatment MERRIL. Once ADHD is diagnosed, regular screening for sleep problems should be performed as a component of ongoing ADHD management [3].

Initial screening should include an exploration of the patient's sleep complaints by way of clinical interview, the use of assessment instruments such as BEARS, and a specific sleep questionnaire such as the Children's Sleep Habits Questionnaire [3]. A written sleep diary or an actigraphy device can be useful for gathering more detailed information about the child's sleep/wake patterns once sleep complaints are endorsed [3]. Other conditions that may cause or contribute to sleep problems should be excluded (See Table 11.1). Disorders such as sleep apnea, and periodic

Table 11.1 Differential diagnoses of sleep disorder symptoms in children with ADHD

Differential Diagnosis	
Potential causes of sleep problems in children with ADHD are as follows:	
Specific sleep disorders	Primary insomnia
	Circadian rhythm sleep disorders, e.g., delayed sleep-wake phase disorder
	Breathing-related sleep disorders, e.g., obstructive sleep apnea and central sleep apnea
	Periodic limb movement disorder
	Parasomnias, e.g., somnambulism, sleep terrors, nightmare disorder, restless legs syndrome
Environmental/behavioral factors	Behavioral insomnia of childhood
	Sleep-onset association type
	Limit-setting type
	Combined type
	Poor sleep hygiene including engaging in sleep-interfering behaviors, e.g., electronic use during sleep time
	Disruptive noise, lights, or extreme temperatures
Psychiatric conditions	ADHD
	Mood disorders (major depressive disorder, dysthymia, bipolar disorder)
	Anxiety disorders (generalized anxiety disorder, separation anxiety)
	Trauma and stressor-related disorders (adjustment disorders, acute stress disorder, post-traumatic stress disorder)
	Psychophysiologic "conditioned" insomnia – heightened physiologic and emotional arousal specifically related to sleep and the sleep environment
	Psychological trauma or stress
	Adjustment to psychosocial stressors
Substance use, abuse, and withdrawal	Caffeine-containing beverages (e.g., colas, coffee, and tea)
	Alcohol
	Tobacco
	Cannabis and synthetic cannabinoids
	Cocaine
	Amphetamines
	Benzodiazepine withdrawal
	Opioid withdrawal

(continued)

Table 11.1 (continued)

Differential Diagnosis	
Potential causes of sleep problems in children with ADHD are as follows:	
Neurological disease	Acquired CNS disorders, e.g., traumatic brain injury, concussion, meningitis, encephalitis, or certain toxic exposures
	Increased intracranial pressure
	Migraines, seizures,
	cerebral palsy, intellectual disability, autism spectrum disorder, sensory blindness associated with neurobehavioral and circadian sleep disruption
Associated medical conditions and their treatments	Obesity
	Pain (acute or chronic)
	Chronic medical disease (e.g., asthma, GERD, anemia, cardiac disease, arthritis, malignancy, or metabolic problems)
Medications	Psychostimulants
	SSRIs
	Anticonvulsants
	Antihistamines
	Corticosteroids
	Diuretics
	Dopamine agonist
	Beta-blockers
	Theophylline
	Thyroid hormone

limb movement disorders when suspected, require polysomnography and referral to a sleep specialist. Other psychiatric conditions associated with sleep difficulties, such as anxiety, and depression commonly co-occur with ADHD [13, 14]. Sleep problems in children or adolescents with comorbid bipolar disorder are six times greater than that in children with ADHD alone [15]. Clinicians should consider these other psychiatric conditions and, if present, their relationship to a child's reported sleep difficulties in order to prioritize treatment strategies [3, 13, 14].

Regular screening for sleep problems should be performed as a component of ongoing ADHD management [16] due to the deleterious effects sleep deficits may have on ADHD symptom control and because ADHD medications themselves, particularly psychostimulants, can negatively impact sleep [2, 11]. Psychostimulant medications such as methylphenidates and amphetamine salts are commonly prescribed for ADHD. Standard practice for ADHD treatment with psychostimulants today may involve administering a long-acting sustained release formulation each morning or immediate release formulations in twice or thrice daily regimes. Often, long-acting and immediate release formulations are used in combination to treat ADHD symptoms during school and after school hours.

Psychostimulants can exacerbate sleep-onset delay greater than 30 minutes, cause sleep phase shift, or make it more difficult to wake in the morning [17]. However, there is considerable variability in their impact on sleep, and study findings differ depending on the study population (e.g., age, comorbidity, whether stimulant naive), dose/dosing schedule, and duration of treatment [7]. Some effects caused by stimulants, such as delayed sleep onset, often occur during titration and for some individuals resolve with time [7]. Sleep disturbances may also be attributed to rebound symptoms of ADHD after the stimulant treatment effect has ceased. Some children experience a "rebound effect" which is an increase in baseline ADHD symptoms occurring during the stimulant medication withdrawal phase [14]. This rebound effect is often worse if the stimulant medication wears off too quickly.

Management of sleep problems in children and adolescents with ADHD should be tailored to the specific conditions underlying the sleep complaint [3, 12]. When patients treated with stimulant medications report insomnia, obtaining a detailed sleep history may clarify whether the onset of insomnia correlates with the initiation of the psychostimulant or pre-dates treatment. Healthy sleep practices, commonly referred to as "sleep hygiene," are modifiable daytime, bedtime, and nighttime practices that have a positive impact on sleep. Evidence-based treatments for behavioral insomnia in typically developing children can be modified for children with ADHD and should be implemented prior to targeted management of specific sleep disorders or conditions and as a first-line option, even if sleep complaints are thought to be medication related [18, 19]. Sleep hygiene practices (such as consistent bed and awakening time or targeting sleep duration according to age-expected norms) have been shown to improve sleep-onset delay in some children with ADHD [8]. While sleep hygiene is a necessary first-line intervention [8, 9], it may not be sufficient for some ADHD children.

If sleep onset difficulties caused by stimulants persist after some weeks (during which time the negative effect of medication on sleep may spontaneously decrease), other options may be considered [9, 20].

When sleep hygiene is not effective, a common strategy is to reduce the total dose or to change the dose regimen or formulation so that less medication is administered later in the day. For example, if the child has insomnia caused by a long-acting methylphenidate medication such as Concerta, an alternative might be to switch to a stimulant medication with a shorter duration of action such as Metadata CD or Ritalin LA. If attempts to stabilize the child's ADHD treatments are still ineffective, one might try changing to a different stimulant (e.g., switching to methylphenidate from amphetamine or vice versa) or to a non-stimulant such as atomoxetine. In some cases, the response to a stimulant has been so robust that the family is reluctant to change medications or has already tried other stimulants which proved ineffective. In such cases, using adjunctive pharmacotherapy might be useful.

There is substantial evidence demonstrating the effectiveness of melatonin in reducing sleep-onset delay in children with ADHD. Specifically, melatonin has been found to advance circadian rhythms of sleep-wake and endogenous melatonin to improve total sleep time in children with ADHD and chronic sleep onset insomnia [21–23].

Open-label studies have reported the efficacy and safety of clonidine in the treatment of ADHD-related sleep disturbances. In some studies, as many as 85% of children treated with clonidine for ADHD-associated sleep disturbances showed significant improvement [24, 25]. A range of other medications such as antihistamine, mirtazapine, clonazepam, trazadone (though there is a risk of priaprism), or mood stabilizers (in the case of treating comorbid bipolar disorder) are used in clinical practice to treat symptoms of insomnia in children with ADHD; however, none have FDA approval, and for the majority of them, information regarding their safety and efficacy is lacking.

If rebound symptoms of ADHD at bedtime interfere with sleep, a combination of stimulants during the day and an alpha-adrenergic agonist in the afternoon, and evening or bedtime can be useful to control the ADHD symptoms [26]. Anecdotal evidence suggests that falling asleep when in rebound from medication is more difficult in some individuals than falling asleep after a low evening dose of stimulant [14]. For this reason, some clinicians will add a third dose of stimulant in the evening if sleep-onset delay is due to a rebound effect.

It can be challenging to determine whether insomnia is due to a direct effect of the stimulant effect, stimulant withdrawal/rebound effect, or a separate sleep disorder. Yet, it is important to distinguish this because the management of insomnia due to direct or indirect effects of stimulants compared to insomnia unrelated to stimulants differs.

Conclusion

In summary, a proper differential diagnosis, assessment of underlying sleep pathology, and treatment of preexisting or co-morbid sleep disorders or conditions are fundamental first steps in managing sleep problems in ADHD children. A detailed sleep history upon initial evaluation of ADHD symptoms, and during management phases, is vital to identifying and addressing sleep issues which might mimic or exacerbate ADHD symptoms and result in functional impairment. Implementing sleep hygiene adapted for ADHD children is a vital component of addressing specific sleep issues prior to utilizing targeted pharmacotherapy. Sleep disturbances are a common side effect of psychostimulant medications, and several pharmacologic options exist for managing stimulant-induced sleep issues. It is important to

Useful Clinical Tips
- Although psychostimulants may cause or exacerbate insomnia in children treated for attention deficit/hyperactivity disorder, an adequate differential diagnosis should also include comorbid sleep disorders and psychiatric conditions.
- Underlying conditions which might negatively impact sleep such as medical conditions, sleep disorders, comorbid psychiatric disorders, or ADHD medications should be appropriately treated.
- Behavioral interventions such as sleep hygiene are first-line treatments for insomnia in children with ADHD, including those with stimulant-induced insomnia.

- If behavioral strategies are not effective for addressing sleep-onset delay caused by ADHD medications, options such as using alternative dosages, dose regimen, formulations, or ADHD medications,
- If a stimulant is necessary, adjunctive medications such as melatonin should be considered to improve sleep.
- Delineating insomnia due to the direct effects of stimulant medications from sleep difficulty due to indirect effects is important as pharmacologic treatment of the two may differ.

elucidate whether sleep difficulties are a result of direct or indirect effects of stimulant, or independent of stimulant treatment, as their management differs.

References

1. Storebo OJ, Ramstad E, Krogh HB, Nilausen TD, Skoog M, Holmskov M, et al. Methylphenidate for children and adolescents with attention deficit hyperactivity disorder (ADHD). Cochrane Database Syst Rev. 2015;(11):CD009885. https://doi.org/10.1002/14651858.CD009885.pub2.
2. Corkum P, Panton R, Ironside S, Macpherson M, Williams T. Acute impact of immediate release methylphenidate administered three times a day on sleep in children with attention-deficit/hyperactivity disorder. J Pediatr Psychol. 2008;33(4):368–79. https://doi.org/10.1093/jpepsy/jsm106.
3. Cortese S, Brown TE, Corkum P, Gruber R, O'Brien LM, Stein M, et al. Assessment and management of sleep problems in youths with attention-deficit/hyperactivity disorder. J Am Acad Child Adolesc Psychiatry. 2013;52(8):784–96. https://doi.org/10.1016/j.jaac.2013.06.001.
4. Sung V, Hiscock H, Sciberras E, Efron D. Sleep problems in children with attention-deficit/hyperactivity disorder: prevalence and the effect on the child and family. Arch Pediatr Adolesc Med. 2008;162(4):336–42. https://doi.org/10.1001/archpedi.162.4.336.
5. Wolraich ML, Wibbelsman CJ, Brown TE, Evans SW, Gotlieb EM, Knight JR, et al. Attention-deficit/hyperactivity disorder among adolescents: a review of the diagnosis, treatment, and clinical implications. Pediatrics. 2005;115(6):1734–46. https://doi.org/10.1542/peds.2004-1959.
6. Cortese S, Faraone SV, Konofal E, Lecendreux M. Sleep in children with attention-deficit/hyperactivity disorder: meta-analysis of subjective and objective studies. J Am Acad Child Adolesc Psychiatry. 2009;48(9):894–908. https://doi.org/10.1097/CHI.0b013e3181ac09c9.
7. Stein MA, Weiss M, Hlavaty L. ADHD treatments, sleep, and sleep problems: complex associations. Neurotherapeutics. 2012;9(3):509–17. https://doi.org/10.1007/s13311-012-0130-0.
8. Vriend J, Corkum P. Clinical management of behavioral insomnia of childhood. Psychol Res Behav Manag. 2011;4:69–79. https://doi.org/10.2147/PRBM.S14057.
9. Waldon J, Vriend J, Davidson F, Corkum P. Sleep and attention in children with ADHD and typically developing peers. J Atten Disord. 2018;22(10):933–41. https://doi.org/10.1177/1087054715575064.
10. Cortese S, Konofal E, Yateman N, Mouren MC, Lecendreux M. Sleep and alertness in children with attention-deficit/hyperactivity disorder: a systematic review of the literature. Sleep. 2006;29(4):504–11.
11. Morash-Conway J, Gendron M, Corkum P. The role of sleep quality and quantity in moderating the effectiveness of medication in the treatment of children with ADHD. Atten Defic Hyperact Disord. 2017;9(1):31–8. https://doi.org/10.1007/s12402-016-0204-7.

12. Konofal E, Lecendreux M, Cortese S. Sleep and ADHD. Sleep Med. 2010;11(7):652–8. https://doi.org/10.1016/j.sleep.2010.02.012.
13. Jensen PS, Hinshaw SP, Kraemer HC, Lenora N, Newcorn JH, Abikoff HB, et al. ADHD comorbidity findings from the MTA study: comparing comorbid subgroups. J Am Acad Child Adolesc Psychiatry. 2001;40(2):147–58. https://doi.org/10.1097/00004583-200102000-00009.
14. Lecendreux M, Cortese S. Sleep problems associated with ADHD: a review of current therapeutic options and recommendations for the future. Expert Rev Neurother. 2007;7(12):1799–806. https://doi.org/10.1586/14737175.7.12.1799.
15. Geller B, Zimerman B, Williams M, Delbello MP, Bolhofner K, Craney JL, et al. DSM-IV mania symptoms in a prepubertal and early adolescent bipolar disorder phenotype compared to attention-deficit hyperactive and normal controls. J Child Adolesc Psychopharmacol. 2002;12(1):11–25. https://doi.org/10.1089/10445460252943533.
16. Cortese S, Holtmann M, Banaschewski T, Buitelaar J, Coghill D, Danckaerts M, et al. Practitioner review: current best practice in the management of adverse events during treatment with ADHD medications in children and adolescents. J Child Psychol Psychiatry. 2013;54(3):227–46. https://doi.org/10.1111/jcpp.12036.
17. Ironside S, Davidson F, Corkum P. Circadian motor activity affected by stimulant medication in children with attention-deficit/hyperactivity disorder. J Sleep Res. 2010;19(4):546–51. https://doi.org/10.1111/j.1365-2869.2010.00845.x.
18. Sciberras E, Mulraney M, Mensah F, Oberklaid F, Efron D, Hiscock H. Sustained impact of a sleep intervention and moderators of treatment outcome for children with ADHD: a randomised controlled trial. Psychol Med. 2019:1–10. https://doi.org/10.1017/S0033291718004063.
19. Hiscock H, Sciberras E, Mensah F, Gerner B, Efron D, Khano S, Oberklaid F. Impact of a behavioural sleep intervention on symptoms and sleep in children with attention deficit hyperactivity disorder, and parental mental health: randomised controlled trial. BMJ. 2015;350:h68. https://doi.org/10.1136/bmj.h68.
20. Cortese S, Lecendreux M, Mouren MC, Konofal E. ADHD and insomnia. J Am Acad Child Adolesc Psychiatry. 2006;45(4):384–5. https://doi.org/10.1097/01.chi.0000199577.12145.bc.
21. Van der Heijden KB, Smits MG, Van Someren EJ, Ridderinkhof KR, Gunning WB. Effect of melatonin on sleep, behavior, and cognition in ADHD and chronic sleep-onset insomnia. J Am Acad Child Adolesc Psychiatry. 2007;46(2):233–41. https://doi.org/10.1097/01.chi.0000246055.76167.0d.
22. Wasdell MB, Jan JE, Bomben MM, Freeman RD, Rietveld WJ, Tai J, et al. A randomized, placebo-controlled trial of controlled release melatonin treatment of delayed sleep phase syndrome and impaired sleep maintenance in children with neurodevelopmental disabilities. J Pineal Res. 2008;44(1):57–64. https://doi.org/10.1111/j.1600-079X.2007.00528.x.
23. Weiss MD, Wasdell MB, Bomben MM, Rea KJ, Freeman RD. Sleep hygiene and melatonin treatment for children and adolescents with ADHD and initial insomnia. J Am Acad Child Adolesc Psychiatry. 2006;45(5):512–9. https://doi.org/10.1097/01chi.0000205706.78818.ef.
24. Prince JB, Wilens TE, Biederman J, Spencer TJ, Wozniak JR. Clonidine for sleep disturbances associated with attention-deficit hyperactivity disorder: a systematic chart review of 62 cases. J Am Acad Child Adolesc Psychiatry. 1996;35(5):599–605. https://doi.org/10.1097/00004583-199605000-00014.
25. Wilens TE, Biederman J, Spencer T. Clonidine for sleep disturbances associated with attention-deficit hyperactivity disorder. J Am Acad Child Adolesc Psychiatry. 1994;33(3):424–6.
26. Kratochvil CJ, Lake M, Pliszka SR, Walkup JT. Pharmacological management of treatment-induced insomnia in ADHD.J. Am Acad Child Adolesc Psychiatry. 2005;44(5):499–501.

Running From Depression: A Case of Antidepressant-Induced Restless Legs Syndrome

Marie-Hélène Rivard and Elliott Kyung Lee

Clinical History/Case

Mrs. Dash, a 73-year-old woman, presents to your office accompanied by her husband. She is referred for consultation by her family physician: "Depressed for past year. Significant insomnia and anxiety. Mirtazapine trial only partially effective. Please provide recommendations regarding treatment of depression for this patient."

Her husband reports that Mrs. Dash has never looked so nervous. She now spends most of the day worrying about her friend who is diagnosed with metastatic lung cancer and her daughter who is in the process of getting a divorce, with the custody of her two children being at the heart of the dispute. Mrs. Dash frequently voices that she feels inadequate for being unable to care for her friend, daughter, and grandchildren. She often cries as she describes these worries to her husband. She has stomach pain, nausea, and constipation, leading to decreased food intake and a 30-pound weight loss in the past 9 months. She appears distracted and has been withdrawing from all social events which are not directly related to caring for her friend or daughter, preferring to rest in bed for hours at a time. Despite feeling "exhausted" throughout the day, she awakens at 4 a.m. daily and is unable to nap during the day. She denies having thoughts of suicide, but endorses passive thoughts of death, adding "when my time comes, I'm okay with sleeping forever."

M.-H. Rivard
Royal Ottawa Mental Health Centre Geriatric Psychiatry Program and University of Ottawa Department of Psychiatry, Ottawa, ON, USA

E. K. Lee (✉)
Royal Ottawa Mental Health Centre Geriatric Psychiatry Program and University of Ottawa Department of Psychiatry, Ottawa, ON, USA

Royal Ottawa Mental Health Centre Sleep Disorders Clinic, Institute for Mental Health Research (IMHR), Ottawa, ON, USA

© Springer Nature Switzerland AG 2021
I. S. Khawaja, T. D. Hurwitz (eds.), *Sleep Disorders in Selected Psychiatric Settings*, https://doi.org/10.1007/978-3-030-59309-4_12

Mrs. Dash has had two prior major depressive episodes at the time of major life transitions. These were effectively treated on an outpatient basis with desipramine (Norpramin). She has never attempted suicide. Her medical history is notable for mild obesity, hypertension, type II diabetes mellitus, and bilateral knee osteoarthritis. These are treated with an angiotensin converting enzyme (ACE) inhibitor, metformin, and acetaminophen PRN. She does not have any allergies. Regarding substance use, she drinks one glass of wine with dinner on weekends and has one cup of coffee every morning. Family history is positive for major depression in her mother and a maternal uncle. There is no family history of sleep disorders.

Four months ago, Mrs. Dash sought care from her GP for these symptoms. She indicated that insomnia and fatigue are her most distressing symptoms, leading her family physician to recommend a trial of mirtazapine, which is currently prescribed at a dose of 30 mg at bedtime. While there has been some decrease in tearfulness and anxiety, she continues to have early-morning insomnia and has now developed difficulties with sleep initiation. Her husband comments: "Doctor, I don't understand… In recent weeks, her sleep is even worse: she can't stop moving her legs in the evening, then she kicks me in her sleep at night! It's almost as though she's trying to run away from this awful depression… Isn't there anything you can do to help her sleep?"

Further inquiry into Mrs. Dash's sleep symptoms reveals that she typically goes to bed at 9 p.m., reads in bed for 1 hour, and readily falls asleep until 6 a.m. the next morning. However, she describes difficulty with sleep maintenance for the past year, with 5 night-time awakenings and an inability to return to sleep after 4 a.m. In the past 4 months, she has been experiencing leg discomfort as she attempts to read in bed. This is accompanied by an urge to move her legs, four or five times a week, and the discomfort is relieved when she walks around or stretches her legs. Her husband reports that she does not typically snore and he has never witnessed any apneas.

Examination/Mental Status Exam

Height: 5'5"	Weight: 185 lbs	BMI: 30.8	Neck circumference: 14"

Vitals: Within normal limits

Cardiovascular: Regular heart rate. Normal S_1 and S_2. No extra heart sounds. No pedal edema.

Respiratory: Good air entry bilaterally. No crackles or wheezing.

Mental Status Exam: Good hygiene. Abdominal obesity. Good eye contact. Alert and cooperative but looks anxious at times and intermittently fidgets during the interview. Soft-spoken. Speech has normal rate and prosody. Organized thought process. No mood-congruent or other delusions elicited. No evidence of perceptual disturbances. Passive suicidal ideation, with no active plan or intent. No aggressive ideations. Fair insight: she acknowledges her symptoms but minimizes the role of depression on her daily functioning. Preserved judgment.

Results

Polysomnography

Technologist's Comments: Periodic limb movements in wakefulness (PLMW) noted prior to sleep onset. Light snoring noted when supine. Patient awoke at 4:13 and was unable to return to sleep.

Total sleep time (TST): 302 minutes

Rapid-eye movement (REM) latency: 43 minutes (pathologically short)

Apnea/hypopnea index (AHI): 3/hour

Respiratory disturbance index (RDI): 7/hour

Periodic limb movements in sleep (PLMS): 42/hour (moderately severe)

PLMS with arousals: 33/hour (moderately severe)

Blood Work

Complete blood count (CBC), electrolytes, creatinine, vitamin B_{12}, and TSH: Within normal limits.

Ferritin: 82 mcg/L.

Questions

1. What is the differential diagnosis for this patient's presentation?
2. Which factors may be contributing to the development of a sleep-related movement disorder for this patient?
3. Which treatment options would you consider for this patient with a comorbid mood disorder and sleep-related movement disorder?

Differential Diagnosis and Diagnosis

Mrs. Dash presents with a one-year history of mood disturbance, as well as a two-month history of motor symptoms at bedtime. Differential diagnosis for this patient includes the following: (1) major depressive disorder, recurrent, moderate to severe and (2) restless legs syndrome (RLS), with periodic limb movement disorder (PLMD). A mood disorder or sleep disorder due to a general medical condition should also be ruled out, although history and investigations thus far do not suggest a physical cause for her symptoms. Similarly, the effects of substance use on her symptoms should be considered. Though the minimal caffeine and alcohol use she describes are unlikely to be the cause of her mood or sleep disorder, the onset of motor symptoms with the initiation of antidepressant treatment suggests the possibility of a medication-induced sleep disorder, as defined in the 5th edition of the Diagnostic and Statistical Manual of Mental Disorders (DSM-5) [1], or of a sleep related movement disorder due to a medication, as defined in the 3rd edition of the International Classification of Sleep Disorders (ICSD-3) [2]. However, when a patient presents with PLMS induced by medication, without RLS, a diagnosis of PLMD is preferred to a general diagnosis of "sleep related movement disorder due to a medication or substance" [2].

Mrs. Dash's symptoms meet full DSM-5 criteria for a major depressive episode with low mood, anhedonia, excessive guilt, poor appetite with weight loss, poor energy, poor concentration, and passive suicidal ideation. She describes the classic depression pattern of early-morning awakening [1]. Her polysomnography reveals decreased REM latency (<50 minutes in elderly patients is considered pathological), a common finding in depressed patients. Other expected polysomnography changes in depressed patients include increased REM density (the number of eye movements per minute of REM sleep), increased time spent in REM sleep, decreased sleep efficiency, increased sleep latency, and increased wake time after sleep onset (WASO) [3]. In contrast, normal sleep changes associated with age include decreased nocturnal total sleep time, delayed onset of sleep, advanced circadian phase, reduced slow-wave sleep, reduced REM sleep, reduced threshold for arousal from sleep, fragmented sleep with multiple arousals, and daytime napping [4].

Mrs. Dash's frequent (four to five times/week) complaints of leg discomfort for the past 4 months are in keeping with a diagnosis of restless legs syndrome, a syndrome of the waking hours. In 2003, Allen et al. proposed four essential criteria for this diagnosis: (1) the patient must experience an urge to move their legs; (2) the urge is worse at rest; (3) the urge is worse in the evening; and finally, (4) the urge is relieved by movement [5]. These criteria form the basis for RLS diagnosis in the DSM-5 and ICSD-3, which also emphasize the importance of ruling out other RLS-mimicking conditions and of considering the level of impairment and distress caused by these symptoms prior to making a formal diagnosis of RLS [1, 2].

The repetitive leg movements observed by Mrs. Dash's husband during her sleep are consistent with periodic limb movements of sleep (PLMS), as supported by the findings on her polysomnography. While over 70% of patients with RLS also have findings of PLMS on polysomnography (70–80% on single-night polysomnography, >90% when multiple nights are recorded), PLMS may also occur in the context of other sleep disorders (REM sleep behavior disorder, narcolepsy and sleep-related breathing disorders) or as a separate entity (periodic limb movement disorder, PLMD) [2]. According to the ICSD-3, a diagnosis of periodic limb movement disorder is given when the PLM index on polysomnography is at least 15/hour, symptoms cause significant impairment or distress, and symptoms are not better explained by another sleep, medical, or mental disorder. Patients experiencing PLMS in the context of RLS should be preferentially diagnosed with RLS. Periodic limb movements can also occur during wakefulness (PLMW) and are thought to be related to RLS [2].

General Remarks

Several factors place Mrs. Dash at increased risk of developing RLS. While the prevalence of RLS is 2–3% in general European and North American populations [2], this is estimated to increase to 10–35% in the elderly population [4]. Similarly, PLMS are common in the elderly and can be observed in approximately 45% of elderly patients [4]. Current diagnostic manuals [1, 2] summarize other protective and risk factors. African and Asian populations have a lower prevalence of the disorder, while women are twice as likely to develop RLS than men. Iron deficiency (ferritin <50–75 mcg/L), pregnancy, chronic renal failure, and uremia are also known as precipitating, exacerbating, and comorbid factors for the disorder. Having a family history of RLS predicts an earlier onset of symptoms (prior to the age of 45–50), while older patients who develop the disorder are less likely to report a family history of RLS. Instead, older patients tend to have a more acute and rapid course of illness, with exacerbating factors also being more common in this population. Cardiovascular disease is the most common medical comorbidity, while depressive, anxiety, and attentional disorders are the most common psychiatric comorbidities [1, 2].

Several medications used in psychiatric care are associated with RLS and/or PLMS (see Table 12.1). Particularly relevant to the practice of psychiatry is the fact that CNS dopamine disturbance and serotoninergic antidepressants are related to RLS [1]. Sedating antihistamines, dopamine receptor antagonists, and most antidepressants – with the exception of bupropion – can also contribute to RLS symptoms [2]. Antidepressants with a strong antihistamine action are often used for their sleep-promoting effects in depressed patients with insomnia, where they are known to decrease sleep latency, increase sleep efficiency, and increase slow-wave sleep. However, antidepressants may also cause unwanted effects on sleep and wakefulness [3]. In a 2017 review article, Wichniak and colleagues examined data from the US Food and Drug Administration (FDA) study register and discussed the effects of various antidepressants on sleep. Reports of daytime somnolence are highest with the sedating antidepressants (mirtazapine 54% vs. 18% placebo; trazodone 46% vs. 19% placebo), though this is also seen with other classes of antidepressants (selective serotonin reuptake inhibitors, SSRI 16% vs. 8% placebo; serotonin-norepinephrine reuptake inhibitors, SNRI 10% vs. 5% placebo). Conversely, while patients rarely report insomnia with mirtazapine (<2%), reports of insomnia with SSRIs and SNRIs are fairly common (SSRI 17% vs. 9% placebo; SNRI 13% vs. 7% placebo) [3].

On history, the onset of Mrs. Dash's RLS symptoms appears to coincide with the initiation of mirtazapine. Several lines of evidence suggest a connection between antidepressant use and RLS/PLMS. In 2005, Yang and colleagues explored the potential link between antidepressant treatment and PLMS on polysomnography in 274 patients treated with antidepressants and 69 controls. Higher rates of PLMS were seen in patients treated with SSRIs and venlafaxine when compared to patients

Table 12.1 Psychotropic medications associated with RLS and/or PLMS

Increased risk of RLS/PLMS	Low risk of RLS/PLMS
Dopamine antagonists	Norepinephrine dopamine reuptake inhibitors
Clozapine	Bupropion[b]
Haldol	Selective norepinephrine reuptake inhibitors
Quetiapine	Reboxetine
Olanzapine	Tricyclic antidepressants
Risperidone	Desipramine[c]
Mood stabilizers	Doxepin
Lithium	Nortriptyline
Serotonin 2 antagonists/reuptake inhibitors	
Trazodone	
Selective serotonin reuptake inhibitors	
Citalopram	
Escitalopram	
Fluoxetine	
Paroxetine	
Sertraline	
Serotonin and norepinephrine reuptake inhibitors	
Duloxetine	
Venlafaxine	
Tetracyclic antidepressants	
Mianserin	
Mirtazapine[a]	
Tricyclic antidepressants	
Clomipramine	
Imipramine	

Compiled from [9, 10, 16–18]. Of note, the current level of evidence supporting the association between medications and RLS/PLMS is limited to case reports and small studies. Data on this topic continues to emerge and may change as larger studies are completed.
[a]Appears to carry the highest risk of RLS/PLMS among antidepressants
[b]May improve RLS/PLMS
[c]Based on adrenergic mechanism of action

who were not treated with antidepressants, while rates were not increased in patients treated with bupropion. The authors concluded that though the clinical significance of these PLMS is unclear, they may affect the tolerability of certain antidepressants [6]. In 2008, Rottach and colleagues explored the link between second-generation antidepressants and RLS. The study included patients treated with fluoxetine, paroxetine, citalopram, sertraline, escitalopram, venlafaxine, duloxetine, reboxetine, and mirtazapine. RLS was most common in patients treated with mirtazapine, with 28% reporting new onset or exacerbation of RLS. In comparison, there were no reported cases of RLS with reboxetine, and RLS was seen in 5–10% of patients treated with the other agents. The authors noticed that RLS symptoms emerged early in the course of treatment, with a median time to onset of 2.5 days and a range of 1–23 days. However, some patients noted decreasing symptoms over time [7]. In 2013, Fulda and colleagues administered mirtazapine to 12 healthy male volunteers aged 20–25 and measured the effects on RLS and PLMS. Eight out of twelve patients demonstrated increased PLMS on polysomnography after the first dose of mirtazapine. Similar to findings by Rottach et al., PLMS emerged on the first night of treatment and tended to dissipate over the 6-day course of follow-up. Three of the twelve patients also experienced temporary RLS symptoms [8]. Kolla, Mansukhani, and Bostwick published a review article focusing on the effects of antidepressants on RLS and PLMS. Overall, 5–9% of patients experienced new onset or worsening of RLS symptoms with SSRIs, though less than 1% of patients reported RLS symptoms spontaneously [9].

In 2005, Picchietti and Winkelman proposed an approach for the treatment of comorbid depression and RLS. Given the frequent comorbidity of these disorders, they recommended assessing all patients with RLS for depression. Treatment recommendations then depend on the severity of the depressive disorder: in cases of mild depression or dysthymia, initial recommendations include treating RLS first and pursuing cognitive psychotherapy and exercise for the depressive symptoms; in more severe cases of depression where an antidepressant is needed, bupropion is recommended as a first choice. If the trial of bupropion is ineffective, a trial of another adrenergic antidepressant such as desipramine or reboxetine is suggested. If this remains ineffective, a serotoninergic medication can be used. Finally, in cases where RLS symptoms persist, Picchietti and Winkelman recommend the addition of RLS treatment. The authors also propose an approach for patients with comorbid depression and RLS who are already on antidepressant treatment. The proposed treatment options include (1) trying a switch to bupropion or desipramine, (2) switching to another antidepressant agent, or (3) decreasing or eliminating the antidepressant [10].

In Mrs. Dash's case, changing mirtazapine to another antidepressant with less likelihood of causing RLS would be in keeping with these recommendations. Bupropion is indicated as a first-line agent for the treatment of major depressive disorder in adults [11, 12] and elderly patients [13]. Given her previous response to desipramine, this medication would also be a reasonable first choice for Mrs. Dash [12]. Should her RLS symptoms persist despite removal of RLS-inducing agents and continue to be disruptive to her sleep, treatment of RLS as a separate entity may be warranted [10]. Current guidelines do not specifically address treatment approaches for medication-induced RLS. The American Academy of Sleep Medicine (AASM) lists pramipexole, ropinirole, and levodopa with a decarboxylase inhibitor and gabapentin enacarbil as the agents with the most evidence for use in the treatment of RLS [14]. Similarly, the International Restless Legs Syndrome Study Group (IRLSSG) suggests that dopamine receptor agonists (such as pramipexole, ropinirole, and rotigotine) and $\alpha_2\delta$ calcium-channel ligands (such as gabapentin enacarbil and pregabalin) can be used as first-line treatments [15]. The presence of certain comorbidities can further guide the choice of agent, with dopamine receptor agonists being preferred in patients who present with comorbid depression, severe symptoms of RLS, increased risk of falls, excess weight, metabolic syndrome, or obstructive sleep apnea. Conversely, $\alpha_2\delta$ calcium-channel ligands may be preferred for patients with comorbid insomnia, painful restless legs, comorbid pain syndromes, history of impulse-control disorders, and comorbid generalized anxiety disorder [15].

For Mrs. Dash, who experienced new-onset RLS symptoms with the initiation of mirtazapine, discontinuation of this medication in favor of an antidepressant with a lower risk of RLS as a side effect is likely to be sufficient to resolve her RLS. In this regard, bupropion or desipramine remains a good choice both for the treatment of depression and to decrease the risks of emergence of RLS during the course of antidepressant treatment. In the unlikely event that symptoms persist, consideration could then be given to augmenting with either pramipexole or gabapentin, but side effect profiles should be taken into account to guide clinical decision-making.

Pearls/Take Home Points
1. RLS and PLMS are potential side effects of most antidepressants with serotoninergic and antihistaminergic effects. Mirtazapine is most commonly associated with RLS and PLMS as side effects, while bupropion is relatively sparing in this regard. Given their similar mechanism of action, other noradrenergic medications may also have less potential for RLS exacerbation.
2. In elderly patients, treatment should start by removing offending agents and addressing underlying medical comorbidities.
3. The addition of medication to treat RLS may be considered if disturbing RLS symptoms persist despite the above, or if a primary diagnosis of RLS is suspected. Patient-specific psychiatric and medical comorbidities may help guide RLS treatment choice toward dopamine receptor agonists or $\alpha_2\delta$ calcium-channel ligands.

References

1. Diagnostic and statistical manual of mental disorders. 5th ed. Arlington: American Psychiatric Association; 2013.
2. International classification of sleep disorders. 3rd ed. Darien: American Academy of Sleep Medicine; 2014.
3. Wichniak A, Wierzbicka A, Walęcka M, Jernajczyk W. Effects of antidepressants on sleep. Curr Psychiatry Rep. 2017;19(9):63. https://doi.org/10.1007/s11920-017-0816-4.
4. Wolkove N, Elkholy O, Baltzan M, Palayew M. Sleep and aging: 1. Sleep disorders commonly found in older people. CMAJ/Journal de l'Association Medicale Canadienne. 2007;176(9):1299–304. https://doi.org/10.1503/cmaj.060792.
5. Allen RP, Picchietti D, Hening WA, Trenkwalder C, Walters AS, Montplaisi J. Restless legs syndrome: diagnostic criteria, special considerations, and epidemiology. Sleep Med. 2003;4(2):101–19. https://doi.org/10.1016/S1389-9457(03)00010-8.
6. Yang C, White DP, Winkelman JW. Antidepressants and periodic leg movements of sleep. Biol Psychiatry. 2005;58(6):510–4. https://doi.org/10.1016/j.biopsych.2005.04.022.
7. Rottach KG, Schaner BM, Kirch MH, Zivotofsky AZ, Teufel LM, Gallwitz T, Messer T. Restless legs syndrome as side effect of second generation antidepressants. J Psychiatr Res. 2008;43(1):70–5. https://doi.org/10.1016/j.jpsychires.2008.02.006.

8. Fulda S, Kloiber S, Dose T, Lucae S, Holsboer F, Schaaf L, Hennings J. Mirtazapine provokes periodic leg movements during sleep in young healthy men. Sleep. 2013;36(5):661–9. https://doi.org/10.5665/sleep.2622.

9. Kolla BP, Mansukhani MP, Bostwick JM. The influence of antidepressants on restless legs syndrome and periodic limb movements: a systematic review. Sleep Med Rev. 2017;38:131. https://doi.org/10.1016/j.smrv.2017.06.002.

10. Picchietti D, Winkelman JW. Restless legs syndrome, periodic limb movements in sleep, and depression. Sleep. 2005;28(7):891–8.

11. Kennedy SH, Lam RW, McIntyre RS, Tourjman SV, Bhat V, Blier P, et al. Canadian Network for Mood and Anxiety Treatments (CANMAT) 2016 clinical guidelines for the management of adults with major depressive disorder: section 3. Pharmacological treatments. Can J Psychiatry. 2016;61(9):540–60. https://doi.org/10.1177/0706743716659417.

12. Gelenberg AJ, Freeman MP, Markowitz JC, Rosenbaum JF, Thase ME, Trivedi MH, Van Rhoads RS. Practice guideline for the treatment of patients with major depressive disorder. 2010. American Psychiatric Association. https://psychiatryonline.org/pb/assets/raw/sitewide/practice_guidelines/guidelines/mdd.pdf.

13. MacQueen GM, Frey BN, Ismail Z, Jaworska N, Steiner M, Lieshout RJV, et al. Canadian Network for Mood and Anxiety Treatments (CANMAT) 2016 clinical guidelines for the management of adults with major depressive disorder: section 6. Special populations: youth, women, and the elderly. Can J Psychiatry. 2016;61(9):588–603. https://doi.org/10.1177/0706743716659276.

14. Aurora RN, Kristo DA, Bista SR, Rowley JA, Zak RS, Casey KR, et al. The treatment of restless legs syndrome and periodic limb movement disorder in adults—an update for 2012: practice parameters with an evidence-based systematic review and meta-analyses. An American Academy of Sleep Medicine Clinical Practice Guideline. Sleep. 2012;35(8):1039–62. https://doi.org/10.5665/sleep.1988.

15. Garcia-Borreguero D, Kohnen R, Silber MH, Winkelman JW, Earley CJ, Högl B, et al. The long-term treatment of restless legs syndrome/Willis–Ekbom disease: evidence-based guidelines and clinical consensus best practice guidance: a report from the International Restless Legs Syndrome Study Group. Sleep Med. 2013;14(7):675–84. https://doi.org/10.1016/j.sleep.2013.05.016.

16. Hornyak M. Depressive disorders in restless legs syndrome: epidemiology, pathophysiology and management. CNS Drugs. 2010;24(2):89–98. https://doi.org/10.2165/11317500-000000000-00000.

17. Cuellar NG. The psychopharmacological management of RLS in psychiatric conditions: a review of the literature. J Am Psychiatr Nurses Assoc. 2012;18(4):214–25. https://doi.org/10.1177/1078390312442569.

18. Koo BB, Blackwell T, Lee HB, Stone KL, Louis ED, Redline S. Restless legs syndrome and depression: effect mediation by disturbed sleep and periodic limb movements. Am J Geriatr Psychiatry. 2016;24(11):1105–16. https://doi.org/10.1016/j.jagp.2016.04.003.

Part VI
Sleep Disturbances in Hospital Setting

Sleep Disturbance During an Acute Manic Episode

13

Melissa Allen, Yasmin Gharbaoui, Chester Wu, Noha Abdel-Gawad, and Mollie Gordon

Clinical History

A 22-year-old woman with no previous psychiatric history presents to the emergency department following an automobile accident. She lost control of her car while speeding at 100 miles per hour late at night while testing her new theory that she is invincible and "cannot be killed." During her evaluation, the patient describes how powerful she is because she has "special DNA" that makes her "more than human." She has slept less than 2 hours of sleep per night seven consecutive days but feels "ready to run a marathon." When asked about the car accident, the patient appears unconcerned and comments about plans to buy a "red Ferrari" when she leaves the hospital.

Collateral information from the patient's mother indicates a family history of bipolar disorder in the maternal aunt. The patient's behavior is an extreme departure from her normal state. According to the family, the patient is typically shy and

M. Allen (✉)
UT Health Harris County Psychiatric Center, Department of Psychiatry and Behavioral Sciences, Houston, TX, USA
e-mail: Melissa.allen@uth.tmc.edu

Y. Gharbaoui
University of Texas Health Science Center at Houston, Department of Psychiatry, Houston, TX, USA

C. Wu
Stanford Health Care, Department of Psychiatry, Redwood City, CA, USA

N. Abdel-Gawad
Inova Fairfax Hospital, Department of Psychiatry, Falls Church, VA, USA

M. Gordon
Ben Taub Hospital, Menninger Department of Psychiatry and Behavioral Sciences, Bellaire, TX, USA

© Springer Nature Switzerland AG 2021
I. S. Khawaja, T. D. Hurwitz (eds.), *Sleep Disorders in Selected Psychiatric Settings*, https://doi.org/10.1007/978-3-030-59309-4_13

conservative, but recently she has been going out every night, spending an exorbitant amount of money, and bringing home strangers.

The patient reports a distant history of trying cocaine 3–4 years ago once and occasionally has three to four drinks when out with friends, but denies any alcohol or drug use in the last month. She stopped smoking cigarettes 2 years ago. She reports attempts to lose weight recently using diet pills, but stopped taking them 3 months ago after they caused her to feel "jittery" and "hyper."

On psychiatric exam, the patient is alert and oriented but appears disheveled. She speaks very rapidly and frequently paces around the room. The patient denies suicidal ideation and any history of self-harm attempts and auditory or visual hallucinations. The patient denies any medical conditions or allergies to medications and is not on any medications at home.

A serum alcohol level and urine drug screen in the emergency department were both negative. Additional medical workup including a head CT, CBC, CMP, TSH, and EKG was all within normal limits.

The on-call psychiatrist diagnoses the patient with bipolar I disorder and most recent episode manic with psychotic features, and admits her to the inpatient psychiatric hospital for further stabilization. After sleeping only 30 minutes the first night, quetiapine 100 mg PO QHS is started and titrated to 200 mg PO QAM and 400 mg PO QHS over the next 6 days.

By hospital day seven, the patient is speaking less rapidly and no longer reports feeling hyper or invincible. She expresses remorse over her recent "reckless behavior," crashing her car, and excessive spending. She still endorses feeling distracted and as if her thoughts are "moving too fast," but this is improving. She is now sleeping about 4 hours a night but was observed by the nursing staff to be napping for 2–3 hours during the day as well.

Discussion Points

- Evaluating the causes and contributing factors of insomnia
- Sleep hygiene techniques and other nonpharmacologic insomnia interventions (Table 13.1)
- Pharmacologic insomnia interventions: the intentional selection of medications to target psychosis and insomnia
- Pharmacologic management of sleep: common mistakes to avoid

Insomnia: Differential Diagnosis

Insomnia is the most common sleeping disorder and, for a sizeable portion of the population, it has a negative impact on quality of life [1]. For this discussion, insomnia is defined as decreased sleep time or quality. Insomnia can be divided into two main categories: short-term insomnia, also referred to as acute insomnia, which usually lasts a few days or weeks, and chronic insomnia, which occurs at least three times per week and persists for at least 3 months [2]. Although the case above reflects an example of acute insomnia secondary to a manic episode, approximately one-third of insomnia cases are of the chronic type [3].

The evaluation of insomnia requires a thorough assessment for secondary causes. Primary insomnia, in which no cause can be identified, only accounts for approximately 25% of cases [4]. The evaluation of secondary causes of insomnias is often approached through broad diagnostic categories: (A) psychiatric causes, (B) medication or substance-induced causes, and (C) medical causes.

A. Insomnia secondary to psychiatric conditions is commonly seen in individuals diagnosed with depressive disorders, bipolar disorders, anxiety disorders, post-traumatic stress disorder, and psychotic disorders. In a study of 7954 participants, Ford and Kamerow [5] found that 40% of those with insomnia had a psychiatric disorder.

In individuals with a current major depressive episode, insomnia symptoms were identified in nearly 80% of the subjects and increased to nearly 90% in individuals with a co-occurring anxiety disorder [6]. The characteristic sleep disturbances seen in major depressive episodes typically include decreased REM latency, reduced sleep efficiency, and loss of the restorative effects of sleep [7]. Early morning awakening can also disturb sleep in depressed individuals [8]. Anxiety disorders are commonly associated with difficulty initiating and maintaining sleep as well as a fragmented sleep pattern on polysomnography. The characteristic sleep disturbances in post-traumatic stress disorder (PTSD) include hypervigilance and nightmares [7].

Short screening instruments such as the Patient Health Questionnaire-2 (PHQ-2), Patient Health Questionnaire-9 (PHQ-9), Generalized Anxiety Disorder 7-item (GAD-7) scale, and Beck Depression Inventory for Primary Care (BDI-PC) can be used to evaluate depression or anxiety in individuals presenting to clinics with a complaint of insomnia. These instruments have the advantage of being brief and can be self-administered by patients before meeting with a clinician. Although these screening tools are not sufficiently accurate to establish a definitive diagnosis for mood or anxiety disorders alone, scores exceeding the threshold for a positive screen should prompt a more thorough diagnostic assessment for mood and/or anxiety disorders [9].

One of the hallmark symptoms of an acute manic or hypomanic episode in individuals with bipolar disorder or schizoaffective disorder is a decreased need for sleep. Sleep disturbances during a manic episode are characterized by extended sleep latency and marked reduction in total sleep time [7]. As in the case vignette, other symptoms of mania will accompany the sleep disturbance and may include increased goal-directed activity, grandiosity, euphoric or irritable mood, and/or pressured speech [10]. In a study examining 3140 individuals with bipolar disorder for triggers of sleep disruption, sleep loss was the most commonly reported trigger of mood episodes, and of those participants, 20% (95% CI 18.6–21.4%, $n = 627$) reported that sleep loss had triggered episodes of mania or hypomania [11]. In addition, an increase in sleep duration may be the first sign of response to the treatment of mania [12]. For these reasons, assessing and treating insomnia are crucial in the treatment and prevention of manic episodes.

B. Use or withdrawal from substances, both illicit and prescribed, can affect sleep dramatically. It is necessary to thoroughly review an individual's current medication list, recent medication changes or discontinuations, over-the-counter medication or herbal supplement use, as well as alcohol, tobacco, or illicit substance use when evaluating insomnia.

Use of activating substances such as caffeine, energy drinks, tobacco, and stimulant medications should be addressed in an insomnia evaluation. Likewise, withdrawal from CNS depressants such as benzodiazepines and alcohol should be evaluated carefully.

The use of alcohol near bedtime accelerates the time to sleep onset, decreases rapid eye movement sleep, and causes sleep disruption in the second half of the sleep period [13]. Revickie, Sobal, and DeForge [14] reported that smokers were more likely to sleep for less than 6 hours per night compared to non-smokers. Similarly, in a sample of 3516 adults, Wetter and Young [15] found that smoking was associated with difficulty initiating sleep and difficulty waking up.

Even common non-psychotropic medications can contribute to insomnia. For example, in an epidemiological study of 8000 Swedish subjects, Bardage and Isacson [16] reported that nearly 20% of the users of anti-hypertensive drugs reported side effects, insomnia being one of those that had the strongest negative impact on health utility.

C. Medical conditions, including sleep disorders and breathing disorders during sleep, can be a major contributor to insomnia and should be ruled out. Important diagnoses to consider when assessing insomnia include sleep apnea, restless legs syndrome, periodic limb movement disorder, circadian rhythm disorders, shift-work disorder, narcolepsy, and parasomnias [17]. Additionally, insomnia can be caused by other common medical conditions such as chronic pain, COPD, cardiovascular disease, thyroid disorders, gastroesophageal reflux disease, neurological disorders, genitourinary conditions, pregnancy, and menopause.

In summary, insomnia is a common and potentially disabling disorder that can occur secondarily to a multitude of conditions. Thorough evaluation for psychiatric, substance-related, and medical causes is vital to the assessment of insomnia. If identified, the treatment of any comorbid disorders should be initiated. In some cases, additional interventions, including both nonpharmacologic techniques and pharmacotherapy, may be indicated.

Sleep Hygiene and Nonpharmacologic Interventions for Insomnia

Sleep disturbance in individuals with bipolar disorder escalates just before a manic or depressive episode, worsens during an episode, and does not always resolve with medication. Even with good adherence to medication, a high proportion of patients with bipolar disorder remain seriously symptomatic in the inter-episode period with clinically significant insomnia being one of the most common residual symptoms. Although the mainstay of treatment for sleep disturbance during acute mania involves pharmacotherapy, there is positive evidence supporting utilization of psychosocial interventions to augment medications during the inter-episode phase of bipolar disorder [18].

Positive evidence has been found for psychoeducation, cognitive behavioral therapy (CBT), family-focused therapy (FFT), interpersonal and social-rhythm therapy (IPSRT), and peer support in the maintenance phase of bipolar disorder. These interventions are included as recommended adjunctive treatment options [19].

A. CBT-I (cognitive behavioral therapy for insomnia), stimulus control, relaxation, and sleep restriction are the standard of care for insomnia [20]. Cognitive therapy for insomnia can be adapted to inpatient unit settings [21]. In manic patients, sleep deprivation is usually due to affective irritability or euphoria rather than anxious worry. Sleep deprivation eventually triggers a period of vast oversleeping (e.g., 12 hours), which subsequently reduces the likelihood of night-time sleep the following night [22].

   CBT-I adaptations may include (1) engagement and assessment, (2) wearable devices, (3) setting sleep windows, (4) stimulus control, (5) targeting hyperarousal with a graded wind down, (6) syncing circadian rhythms, (7) reducing nighttime exposures, (8) working with distressing experiences at night, and (9) managing discharge as a challenge for sleep.

   Group cognitive behavioral therapy (G-CBT) may be adapted to the inpatient unit. In outpatient studies of primary care patients with insomnia, fatigue severity, mood, health-related quality of life, general daytime functioning, specific daytime symptoms, and dysfunctional beliefs improved with nurse-led groups [23].

B. Social rhythm therapy has been shown to provide a potentially useful model for managing mania in the inpatient setting [24]. Social rhythm therapy consists of sleep and circadian regulation focusing on the establishment and maintenance of regular daily rhythms, particularly in relation to sleep-wake times, meal times, and socialization. In a study randomizing manic patients to a trial of IPSRT to Intensive Case Management (ICM) as additive to pharmacological interventions, IPSRT in the acute phase of treatment reduced the risk of recurrence regardless of maintenance treatment [25].

   Inpatient schedules can help maintain healthy sleep-wake schedules. For example, staff may awaken patients at a regular hour with the opportunity for exposure to daylight on awakening. Patients should be encouraged to eat regular meals, especially breakfast, and structure time for socialization. During groups and therapy, patients should be in the milieu, while the rooms should be used only for sleep (stimulus control therapy). Minimum time in quiet, dark rooms should be set to 6 hours.

C. Rooms may be modified to mitigate insomnia. A specialized sensory room with items to relax and perform self-soothing routines can be made available. The most common activities used by acute inpatients (where a quarter of the usage was by manic patients) were use of a weighted blanket, listening to music, reading, and a rocking chair [26].

Additionally, patients may participate in dark room therapy. In a study randomizing 14 hours of dark room therapy for 3 days in inpatient manic patients, results illustrated an improvement in mania scores by 50%, nearly 9 days earlier discharge, and lower pharmacotherapy use for patients who had been receiving treatment for less than 2 weeks. It is theorized that when dark therapy is used early in mania, sleep-wake rhythms can be stabilized to prevent sleep-loss triggering mania [27].

D. Inpatient hospitalization also offers an opportunity for family involvement and psychoeducation on the importance of sleep hygiene and recognizing changes in sleep patterns as early warning signs of decompensation [28].

Pharmacologic Management of Insomnia During an Acute Manic Episode

There are many pharmacologic considerations in the treatment of insomnia. This section specifically addresses the treatment of insomnia during an acute manic episode, as described in the clinical vignette. Prior to initiating pharmacologic treatment for insomnia, any current activating medications should be reduced in dose or discontinued as appropriate. If not possible, efforts should be made to administer these medications as soon as patients wake up in order to minimize their plasma concentrations during sleep hours. If a patient in a manic episode is receiving antidepressant treatment, the risks versus benefits of ongoing use should be thoroughly reviewed as serotonergic medications may exacerbate manic symptoms [29].

The American Psychiatric Association guidelines for treating mild to moderate mania or hypomania state that monotherapy with lithium, valproic acid, and antipsychotics is equally efficacious [30]. When targeting insomnia, preference should be given to sedating antipsychotics such as quetiapine or olanzapine unless otherwise contraindicated. Of the FDA-approved medications for treating mania, the

Table 13.1 Sleep Hygiene Tips for Managing Insomnia

Sleep hygiene tips for chronic insomnia
Avoid napping during the day
Maintain a consistent time for waking and going to sleep daily, including weekends
Avoid using the bed for activities other than sleep such as reading or watching TV
Minimize lights and electronics in the bedroom
Limit caffeine intake to less than 200 mg daily and avoid consuming caffeine after lunch
If unable to fall asleep within 20 minutes, get out of bed and use a relaxation technique. Return to bed when feeling drowsy
Discontinue or reduce consumption of alcoholic beverages
Decrease evening stimulation
Avoid smoking, especially in the evening

three most efficacious medications were found to be risperidone, haloperidol, and olanzapine. The three best tolerated medications of the same group were olanzapine, risperidone, and quetiapine [31]. Of note, though aripiprazole is FDA-approved in the treatment of acute mania, it has been shown to have activating effects in some patients and may therefore be less efficacious when specifically targeting insomnia [32]. When choosing between valproic acid and lithium (e.g., in the setting of sensitivity to extrapyramidal symptoms), one should consider that valproic acid exhibits stronger sedative effects compared to lithium. Therefore, it may be more potent in the treatment of insomnia [32]. No studies exist directly comparing the sedating effects of lithium or valproate versus antipsychotics.

In the case of severe mania, evidence supports first-line treatment with combination pharmacotherapy using lithium and an antipsychotic or valproic acid and an antipsychotic [30]. Given that valproic acid causes more sedation than lithium at therapeutic doses [32], it may be preferable to combine valproic acid with a second-generation antipsychotic.

In patients with preexisting bipolar disorder who are already on psychotropic medications, optimization of dosing should take priority over changing medications. This can be done by increasing the dosage of any mood stabilizers, including antipsychotics. Given the quick onset of sedating properties of many of these drugs, split-dosing regimens should favor a higher dose at bedtime, while maintaining a therapeutic total daily dose.

If these changes are insufficient, insomnia is severe, or the patient is agitated, a short course of benzodiazepines may be indicated [19]. Clonazepam and lorazepam have been widely studied and found to be effective in reducing sleep onset and increasing total sleep time. A 2002 meta-analysis of seven randomized controlled trials comparing clonazepam or lorazepam monotherapy to placebo, haloperidol, or lithium in the treatment of acute mania found that clonazepam was comparable to haloperidol and lithium in its efficacy [33]. However, given their potential for toxicity and abuse, monotherapy with benzodiazepines is not first line. The American Psychiatric Association practice guidelines recommend using benzodiazepines as short-term adjunct therapy [30]. The need for benzodiazepines should be reassessed frequently and discontinued once symptoms improve. As further explained, benzodiazepines are not recommended to be used longer than 4 weeks [20]. In patients with concurrent substance use disorders or in whom benzodiazepines are contraindicated, alternatives such as benzodiazepine receptor agonists (BZRAs; e.g., zolpidem, zaleplon, and eszopiclone) may be particularly useful. BZRAs, like benzodiazepines, target GABA-A receptors. However, they have shorter half-lives and their action is more specific at the alpha-1 subunit of said receptors, mitigating their anxiolytic effect and reducing their potential for abuse, tolerance, withdrawal, daytime sedation, and motor/cognitive impairment compared to benzodiazepines [34]. These agents, like their benzodiazepine counterparts, should be discontinued as early as possible.

Other popular drugs used as hypnotics in mania include anticonvulsants due to their sedating effects and mood-stabilizing properties, despite the lack of FDA approval for the treatment of bipolar disorder. These include gabapentin and topiramate. Gabapentin has been suggested to increase REM and slow-wave sleep as well as to increase subjective sleep quality [35]. Melatonin and melatonin receptor agonists such as ramelteon may also be useful due to their very low potential for abuse [36]. Melatonin has also been shown to have some efficacy as adjunctive pharmacotherapy in treatment-refractory mania in rapid cycling patients [37].

Clinical Pearls

A. Careful and measured use of benzodiazepines is essential when being prescribed for insomnia. Some are in favor of limiting benzodiazepines to emergency situations where a rapid symptomatic amelioration is required [38], such as in the patient in the clinical vignette. That said, benzodiazepines are intended to be used for no more than 4 weeks in the treatment of severe anxiety or insomnia that is resistant to multiple evidence-based treatments [20]. Despite recommendations against long-term benzodiazepine use, many providers continue to prescribe them for months or years, allowing for dependence and diversion [39]. Inpatient psychiatric treatment is one of many factors increasing the likelihood of an individual being prescribed benzodiazepines [40]. It is therefore essential to consider the chronicity of insomnia prior to starting benzodiazepine initiation and reassess sleep and hypnotic necessity prior to discharge.

There is evidence that even short-term use of benzodiazepines can decrease sleep time, decrease deep-stage/slow-wave sleep, increase rapid eye movement (REM) sleep latency, increase stage 2 non-REM sleep, and decrease slow-wave sleep [41]. However, these sleep changes are not permanent and sleep parameters will improve following benzodiazepine discontinuation after an initial rebound of insomnia during withdrawal [41].

Benzodiazepine use disorder with prescribed medications occurs in at least 50% of patients with preexisting or active substance use disorders [39]. Except in cases of acute alcohol or sedative hypnotic withdrawal, benzodiazepines are contraindicated for patients with any history of substance use disorders [20].

Benzodiazepines can cause paradoxical reactions including disinhibition, impulsivity, excitement, irritability, aggression, hostility, rage attacks, violence, or homicidal and suicidal ideations [42]. The theorized mechanism of action is pre-frontal cortex disinhibition and systemic inhibition of serotonin [43]. Additionally, while the anxiolytic and hypnotic effects of benzodiazepines disappear as tolerance develops, anger and impulsivity with high suicidal risk may persist [44]. This makes differentiating the underlying bipolar disorder from the secondary effects of benzodiazepine use difficult.

B. The use of a combination of antipsychotics is not recommended in patients with mania. As previously mentioned, the American Psychiatric Association recommends a combination of lithium or valproic acid with an antipsychotic to treat mania with psychotic features [30]. Monotherapy with an antipsychotic can also be considered for less severe mania or hypomania.

The most common scenario in which a patient might be prescribed a combination of antipsychotics is in treatment-refractory schizophrenia. Studies have suggested prevalence of combination antipsychotics in patients with schizophrenia to be approximately 19.6% worldwide [45]. According to the Joint Commission's Hospital-Based Inpatient Psychiatric Services measures [46], combination antipsychotic treatment is only justified if there is documentation of three failed trials of monotherapy, a plan to taper/cross-taper to monotherapy, and augmentation of clozapine.

The most common concerns of combination antipsychotic use are higher risk of side effects [47], pharmacokinetic interactions, and increased cost. Furthermore, studies have not consistently demonstrated improved outcomes or increased efficacy with combination antipsychotic therapy for schizophrenia compared to monotherapy. No studies have been performed on the utility of combination antipsychotic use to treat acute mania.

C. With the prevalence and desperation of patients with insomnia, patients and providers should be conscientious of sleep aid polypharmacy and misuse. Studies have demonstrated at least 10% of patients have used some type of medication to fall asleep in the preceding year [48]. One study found that in 2009–2010, 3.5% of patients reported being prescribed a medication for insomnia in the previous month. A total of 55% of these patients were concurrently receiving at least one other sedating medication and 10% were taking more than three other sedating medications [49].

Many patients with sleep disturbances do not consult with their doctor and often self-medicate with over-the-counter supplements such as antihistamines (doxylamine, diphenhydramine), melatonin, or substances such as alcohol and marijuana/cannabidiol. In a study of 2000 adult Canadians, 9.0% used natural products, 5.7% used over-the-counter products, and 4.6% used alcohol as sleep aids in the previous year [50]. A 1996 study of the Detroit population found that 13% of subjects used alcohol, 18% used medications, and 5% used both as sleep aids in the previous year [51].

D. As previously mentioned, insomnia can occur as a result of many factors including psychiatric and medical disorders, medications, substance use, or other sleep disorders. It is therefore essential to consider other precipitating and perpetuating factors of insomnia. In these cases, the treatment of insomnia begins with the identification and treatment of the underlying condition. Therefore, a thorough history, medication reconciliation, and prompt referral to other providers should be performed as needed.

E. Before initiating pharmacotherapy for insomnia, providers should adequately educate patients on treatment options including psychological and behavioral therapies, and establish treatment goals and expectations. Hypnotics, if used, are typically recommended to be of short term and supplemented by nonpharmacological therapy. Safety concerns, potential for side effects and drug interactions, potential for dosage escalation, and rebound insomnia should be discussed with patients [52]. Close follow-up including review of effectiveness, adverse effects, and need for continued medication should be conducted regularly.

Summary

Insomnia is commonly encountered in psychiatric patients. It is essential for the practitioner to identify potential precipitants and contributing factors to insomnia including psychiatric disorders, medical disorders, sleep disorders, medications, and substance use. In acute insomnia, due to these conditions, treatment begins with the management of the underlying issues. Nonpharmacological therapies including CBT-I and sleep hygiene should be incorporated early and throughout insomnia treatment as pharmacotherapy, particularly chronic use, is not recommended.

References

1. Léger D, Bayon V. Societal costs of insomnia. Sleep Med Rev. 2010;14(6):379–89. https://doi.org/10.1016/j.smrv.2010.01.003.
2. American Academy of Sleep Medicine. International classification of sleep disorders. 3rd ed. Darien: American Academy of Sleep Medicine; 2014.
3. American Academy of Sleep Medicine. Fact sheet for insomnia. 2008. Retrieved from https://aasm.org/resources/factsheets/insomnia.pdf.
4. Doghramji K. The epidemiology and diagnosis of insomnia. Am J Manag Care. 2006;12(Supplement 8):S214–20. https://www.ajmc.com/journals/supplement/2006/2006-05-vol12-n8suppl/may06-2307ps214-s220?p=2.
5. Ford DE, Kamerow DB. Epidemiologic study of sleep disturbances and psychiatric disorders. JAMA. 1989;262(11):1479–84. https://doi.org/10.1001/jama.1989.03430110069030.
6. Ohayon MM, Shapiro CM, Kennedy SH. Differentiating DSM-IV anxiety and depressive disorders in the general population: comorbidity and treatment consequences. Can J Psychiatry. 2000;45(2):166–72. https://doi.org/10.1177/070674370004500207.
7. Kaufman DM. Clinical neurology for psychiatrists. 6th ed. Philadelphia: Saunders; 2007.
8. Sadock BJ, Sadock VA, Ruiz P. Kaplan & Sadock's synopsis of psychiatry: behavioral sciences/clinical psychiatry. 11th ed. Philadelphia: Wolter Kluwer/Lippincott Williams & Wilkins; 2015.
9. Mitchell AJ, Coyne JC. Do ultra-short screening instruments accurately detect depression in primary care? Br J Gen Pract. 2007;57(535):144–51. Retrieved from https://bjgp.org/content/57/535/144.long.
10. Diagnostic and statistical manual of mental disorders. 5th ed. 2013. Arlington: American Psychiatric Publishing.
11. Lewis KS, Gordon-Smith K, Forty L, Florio AD, Craddock N, Jones L, Jones I. Sleep loss as a trigger of mood episodes in bipolar disorder: individual differences based on diagnostic subtype and gender. Br J Psychiatry. 2017;211(3):169–74. https://doi.org/10.1192/bjp.bp.117.202259.
12. Galynker II, Yaseen ZS, Koppolu SS, Vaughan B, Szklarska-Imiolek M, Cohen LJ, et al. Increased sleep duration precedes the improvement of other symptom domains during the treatment of acute mania: a retrospective chart review. BMC Psychiatry. 2016;16(1):1–9. https://doi.org/10.1186/s12888-016-0808-7.
13. Colrain IM, Nicholas CL, Baker FC. Alcohol and the sleeping brain. Handb Clin Neurol. 2014;125:415–31. https://doi.org/10.1016/b978-0-444-62619-6.00024-0.
14. Revicki D, Sobal J, DeForge B. Smoking status and the practice of other unhealthy behaviors. Fam Med. 1991;23(5):361–4.
15. Wetter DW, Young TB. The relation between cigarette smoking and sleep disturbance. Prev Med. 1994;23(3):328–34. https://doi.org/10.1006/pmed.1994.1046.

16. Bardage C, Isacson DG. Self-reported side-effects of antihypertensive drugs: an epidemiological study on prevalence and impact on health-state utility. Blood Press. 2000;9(6):328–34. https://doi.org/10.1080/080370500300000905.
17. Gupta R, Zalai D, Spence DW, Bahammam AS, Ramasubramanian C, Monti JM, Pandi-Perumal SR. When insomnia is not just insomnia: the deeper correlates of disturbed sleep with reference to DSM-5. Asian J Psychiatr. 2014;12:23–30. https://doi.org/10.1016/j.ajp.2014.09.003.
18. Harvey AG, Kaplan KA, Soehner AM. Interventions for sleep disturbance in bipolar disorder. Sleep Med Clin. 2015;10(1):101–5. https://doi.org/10.1016/j.jsmc.2014.11.005.
19. Yatham LN, Kennedy SH, Parikh SV, Schaffer A, Bond DJ, Frey BN, et al. Canadian Network for Mood and Anxiety Treatments (CANMAT) and International Society for Bipolar Disorders (ISBD) 2018 guidelines for the management of patients with bipolar disorder. Bipolar Disord. 2018;20(2):97–170. https://doi.org/10.1111/bdi.12609.
20. Guina J, Merrill B. Benzodiazepines I: upping the care on downers: the evidence of risks, benefits and alternatives. J Clin Med. 2018;7(2):17. https://doi.org/10.3390/jcm7020017.
21. Sheaves B, Isham L, Bradley J, Espie C, Barrera A, Waite F, et al. Adapted CBT to stabilize sleep on psychiatric wards: a transdiagnostic treatment approach. Behav Cogn Psychother. 2018;46(6):661–75. https://doi.org/10.1017/s1352465817000789.
22. Sheaves B, Freeman D, Isham L, Mcinerney J, Nickless A, Yu L, et al. Stabilising sleep for patients admitted at acute crisis to a psychiatric hospital (OWLS): an assessor-blind pilot randomised controlled trial. Psychol Med. 2018;48(10):1694–704. https://doi.org/10.1017/s0033291717003191.
23. Sandlund C, Hetta J, Nilsson GH, Ekstedt M, Westman J. Impact of group treatment for insomnia on daytime symptomatology: analyses from a randomized controlled trial in primary care. Int J Nurs Stud. 2018;85:126–35. https://doi.org/10.1016/j.ijnurstu.2018.05.002.
24. Crowe M, Porter R. Inpatient treatment for mania: a review and rationale for adjunctive interventions. Aust N Z J Psychiatry. 2014;48(8):716–21. https://doi.org/10.1177/0004867414540754.
25. Frank E, Kupfer DJ, Thase ME, Mallinger AG, Swartz HA, Fagiolini AM, et al. Two-year outcomes for interpersonal and social rhythm therapy in individuals with bipolar I disorder. Arch Gen Psychiatry. 2005;62(9):996–1004. https://doi.org/10.1001/archpsyc.62.9.996.
26. Novak T, Scanlan J, Mccaul D, Macdonald N, Clarke T. Pilot study of a sensory room in an acute inpatient psychiatric unit. Australas Psychiatry. 2012;20(5):401–6. https://doi.org/10.1177/1039856212459585.
27. Barbini B, Benedetti F, Colombo C, Dotoli D, Bernasconi A, Cigala-Fulgosi M, et al. Dark therapy for mania: a pilot study. Bipolar Disord. 2005;7(1):98–101. https://doi.org/10.1111/j.1399-5618.2004.00166.x.
28. Pon NC, Gordon MR, Coverdale J, Nguyen PT. Content-area framework for conducting family meetings for acutely ill psychiatric patients. J Psychiatr Pract. 2016;22(5):416–21. https://doi.org/10.1097/pra.0000000000000176.
29. Tondo L, Vázquez G, Baldessarini RJ. Mania associated with antidepressant treatment: comprehensive meta-analytic review. Acta Psychiatr Scand. 2010;121(6):404–14. https://doi.org/10.1111/j.1600-0447.2009.01514.x.
30. Hirschfeld RM, Bowden CL, Gitlin MJ, Keck PE, Suppes T, Thase ME, et al. Practice guideline for the treatment of patients with bipolar disorder. APA practice guidelines for the treatment of psychiatric disorders: comprehensive guidelines and guideline watches. 2002. https://doi.org/10.1176/appi.books.9780890423363.50051.
31. Yildiz A, Nikodem M, Vieta E, Correll CU, Baldessarini RJ. A network meta-analysis on comparative efficacy and all-cause discontinuation of antimanic treatments in acute bipolar mania. Psychol Med. 2015;45(2):299–317. https://doi.org/10.1017/s0033291714001305.
32. Stahl SM. Prescriber's guide: Stahl's essential psychopharmacology. 5th ed. New York: Cambridge University Press; 2014.
33. Curtin F, Schulz P. Clonazepam and lorazepam in acute mania: a Bayesian meta-analysis. J Affect Disord. 2004;78(3):201–8. https://doi.org/10.1016/s0165-0327(02)00317-8.

34. Plante DT, Winkelman JW. Sleep disturbance in bipolar disorder: therapeutic implications. Am J Psychiatry. 2008;165(7):830–43. https://doi.org/10.1176/appi.ajp.2008.08010077.
35. Foldvary-Schaefer N, De Leon Sanchez I, Karafa M, Mascha E, Dinner D, Morris H. Gabapentin increases slow-wave sleep in normal adults. Epilepsia. 2002;43(12):1493–7. https://doi.org/10.1046/j.1528-1157.2002.21002.x.
36. Griffiths RR, Johnson MW. Relative abuse liability of hypnotic drugs: a conceptual framework and algorithm for differentiating among compounds. J Clin Psychiatry. 2005;66(Supplement 9):31–41. Retrieved from https://www.psychiatrist.com/jcp/article/Pages/2005/v66s09/v66s0906.aspx.
37. Bersani G, Garavini A. Melatonin add-on in manic patients with treatment resistant insomnia. Prog Neuropsychopharmacol Biol Psychiatry. 2000;24(2):185–91. https://doi.org/10.1016/s0278-5846(99)00097-4.
38. Bourin M, Lambert O. Pharmacotherapy of anxious disorders. Hum Psychopharmacol Clin Exp. 2002;17(8):383–400. https://doi.org/10.1002/hup.435.
39. Ashton H. The diagnosis and management of benzodiazepine dependence. Curr Opin Psychiatry. 2005;18(3):249–55. https://doi.org/10.1097/01.yco.0000165594.60434.84.
40. Kosten TR, Fontana A, Sernyak MJ, Rosenheck R. Benzodiazapine use in posttraumatic stress disorder among veterans with substance abuse. J Nerv Ment Dis. 2000;188(8):454–9. Retrieved from https://pdfs.semanticscholar.org/e774/0defc4683785e0c8edfd0f6101f14217f237.pdf.
41. Poyares D, Guilleminault C, Ohayon MM, Tufik S. Chronic benzodiazepine usage and withdrawal in insomnia patients. J Psychiatr Res. 2004;38(3):327–34. https://doi.org/10.1016/j.jpsychires.2003.10.003.
42. Jones KA, Nielsen S, Bruno R, Frei M, Lubman DI. Benzodiazepines: their role in aggression and why GPs should prescribe with caution. Aust Fam Physician. 2011;40(11):862–5. Retrieved from https://www.racgp.org.au/download/documents/AFP/2011/November/201111jones.pdf.
43. Saleh FM, Fedoroff JP, Ahmed AG, Pinals DA. Treatment of violent behavior. Psychiatry. 2008;3:2603–15. https://doi.org/10.1002/9780470515167.ch127.
44. Michelini S, Cassano GB, Frare F, Perugi G. Long-term use of benzodiazepines: tolerance, dependence and clinical problems in anxiety and mood disorders. Pharmacopsychiatry. 1996;29(04):127–34. https://doi.org/10.1055/s-2007-979558.
45. Gallego JA, Bonetti J, Zhang J, Kane JM, Correll CU. Prevalence and correlates of antipsychotic polypharmacy: a systematic review and meta-regression of global and regional trends from the 1970s to 2009. Schizophr Res. 2012;138(1):18–28. https://doi.org/10.1016/j.schres.2012.03.018.
46. The Joint Commission. Appropriate justification for multiple antipsychotic medications. Specifications manual for joint commission national quality measures (v2017B2). 2017. Retrieved from https://manual.jointcommission.org/releases/TJC2017B2/DataElem0137.html.
47. Gallego JA, Nielsen J, De Hert M, Kane JM, Correll CU. Safety and tolerability of antipsychotic polypharmacy. Expert Opin Drug Saf. 2012;11(4):527–42. https://doi.org/10.1517/14740338.2012.683523.
48. Vaidya V, Gabriel MH, Gangan N, Borse M. Characteristics of prescription and nonprescription sleep medication users in the United States. Popul Health Manag. 2014;17(6):345–50. https://doi.org/10.1089/pop.2013.0124.
49. Bertisch SM, Herzig SJ, Winkelman JW, Buettner C. National use of prescription medications for insomnia: NHANES 1999–2010. Sleep. 2014;37(2):343–9. https://doi.org/10.5665/sleep.3410.
50. Morin CM, Leblanc M, Bélanger L, Ivers H, Mérette C, Savard J. Prevalence of insomnia and its treatment in Canada. Can J Psychiatry. 2011;56(9):540–8. https://doi.org/10.1177/070674371105600905.
51. Johnson EO, Roehrs T, Roth T, Breslau N. Epidemiology of alcohol and medication as aids to sleep in early adulthood. Sleep. 1998;21(2):178–86. https://doi.org/10.1093/sleep/21.2.178.
52. Schutte-Rodin S, Broch L, Buysse D, Dorsey C, Sateia M. Clinical guideline for the evaluation and management of chronic insomnia in adults. J Clin Sleep Med. 2008;4(5):487–504. Retrieved from https://www.ncbi.nlm.nih.gov/pmc/articles/PMC2576317/.

Sleep in the ICU

14

Adam N. Young, John C. Hunninghake, Aaron B. Holley, and Robert J. Walter

Introduction

Disruption in normal sleep patterns is a common experience during illness, particularly during periods of prolonged or severe sickness. Additionally, even healthy individuals may experience difficulty sleeping in unfamiliar environments due to a variety of factors (i.e., travel, time change, temperature, different sounds, different rooms, or bedding). Combining the normal stressors affecting sleep when in an unfamiliar setting with those of critical illness and the inpatient hospital environment frequently leads to a significant disruption of the circadian cycle and sleep efficiency as well as a diminishment in the restorative effects of sleep.

Clinical History/Case

A 54-year-old male with a past medical history significant for obesity, hypertension, diabetes mellitus type II, and chronic kidney disease presents to the emergency department (ED) febrile with cough and progressive dyspnea over the past week.

A. N. Young
Kadena Medical Group/U.S. Navy Hospital Okinawa, Critical Care Air Transport/Intensive Care Unit, APO, AP, Japan

J. C. Hunninghake · R. J. Walter (✉)
Brooke Army Medical Center, Department of Pulmonary/Critical Care Medicine, JBSA Fort Sam Houston, TX, USA
e-mail: robert.j.walter26.mil@mail.mil

A. B. Holley
Walter Reed National Military Medical Center, Department of Pulmonary and Critical Care Medicine, Bethesda, MD, USA

© Springer Nature Switzerland AG 2021
I. S. Khawaja, T. D. Hurwitz (eds.), *Sleep Disorders in Selected Psychiatric Settings*, https://doi.org/10.1007/978-3-030-59309-4_14

His vital signs at triage are T 39.2°C, HR 108, BP 134/72 mmHg, RR 20, SpO$_2$ 91% on room air. A portable chest X-ray demonstrates a faint right upper lobe opacity, and laboratory studies are significant for a leukocytosis of 18,000 cells/μL and eGFR of 40 mL/min. Respiratory and blood cultures are obtained in the ED before starting antibiotics (ceftriaxone and azithromycin), and the patient is admitted to the intermediate care unit for continuous telemetry and pulse oximetry monitoring.

The patient's viral respiratory panel is positive for influenza type A H3N2, and he is started on oseltamivir. Blood cultures remain negative, and his antibiotics are discontinued. Despite antiviral therapy and supportive care, he has worsening tachypnea and hypoxemia. He is trialed on non-invasive positive pressure ventilation (NIPPV) before ultimately being intubated for respiratory failure and transferred to the medical intensive care unit (MICU) for continued management. A repeat chest roentgenogram (CXR) following intubation demonstrates appropriate placement of the endotracheal tube and new bilateral infiltrates. An arterial blood gas (ABG) is obtained which reveals a respiratory acidosis with a pH 7.2, PaCO$_2$ 80 mmHg, PaO$_2$ 120 mmHg, and FiO$_2$ 1.0. He does not appear to be in acute heart failure and his PaO$_2$/FiO$_2$ ratio is 120. He is initiated on lung-protective ventilator settings, and his antibiotics are restarted and broadened to vancomycin and piperacillin-tazobactam with the continuation of oseltamivir. He requires intermittent fluid boluses and vasopressor support with norepinephrine to maintain MAP higher than 65 mmHg.

His CXR progressively worsens and he continues to have periodic fevers. During an unusually high fever episode (40°C), the patient has a convulsive seizure which abates with rapid cooling and lorazepam 4 mg IV. His sedation is transitioned to propofol and antibiotic coverage is further broadened to meropenem. Itraconazole is also added for empiric antifungal coverage given his history of diabetes. A post-seizure non-contrasted CT of the head did not demonstrate evidence of an acute intracranial pathologic process. A subsequent lumbar puncture is negative for bacterial and viral meningitis by polymerase chain reaction amplification. He remains sedated and is placed on continuous electroencephalography (EEG) monitoring without additional convulsive episodes. EEG shows diffuse slowing (low-voltage, low-frequency, slow-wave activity) and is unchanged when sedation is held.

Examination/Mental Status Exam

Current vitals: height 68 in, weight 113 kg, BMI 38 kg/m^2, T 37.8°C, HR 112, BP 90/54 mmHg (MAP 66 mmHg), RR 18

Ventilator settings: pressure control (PC) mode, respiratory rate 15 breaths per minute, inspiratory pressure (PHi) 28 cm H$_2$O, positive end expiratory pressure (PEEP) 14 cm H$_2$O, FiO$_2$ 0.9 (average tidal volume 380 ml [5–6 ml/kg])

Upon exam, you observe an obese male resting supine in the bed with head inclined to 30 degrees. He is orally intubated and has an oral-gastric tube in place. He is on a norepinephrine drip to maintain MAP goals and is sedated on propofol and fentanyl continuous infusions with a Richmond agitation-sedation scale (RASS) score of −2. He appears comfortable and is synchronous with the ventilator. He is rousable to voice but unable to sustain eye contact for more than a few seconds and does not follow commands. Pupils are constricted but equal and reactive. When sedation is reduced, he becomes agitated and asynchronous with the ventilator. His exam is significant for bilateral breath sounds with fine rales and occasional expiratory wheezes. He is tachycardic with normal S1 and S2 heart sounds. There are no murmurs, rubs, or gallops, and he has 2+ dependent edema. His abdomen is large and protuberant. Bowel sounds are present but diminished, and his abdomen is soft without apparent guarding or tenderness. There are soft restraints on his upper extremities, and he has spontaneous movement of both upper and lower extremities when sedation is lightened. Bilateral reflexes are intact and within normal limits.

Questions

- *What environmental factors are affecting patients' sleep at this time, and how can I improve these factors?*

  Sleep disruption within the hospital environment and its effects on patient recovery is a growing area of focus as medicine has evolved into a more patient-centered model. Several general strategies have been proposed to facilitate sleep in the ICU environment [1, 2]. Most of these strategies highlight similar core environmental issues like lighting, noise, intrusive monitoring, patient care, and procedures that routinely affect the quantity and quality of patient sleep in the hospital.

  Hospitals have traditionally been designed with the primary intent to facilitate efficient and effective patient care. To this end, lighting levels are configured to allow optimal visualization during patient encounters and help prevent falls. While lighting is necessary for patient care and safety, attempts to prevent disruption in the normal sleep-wake circadian cycle due to intrusive nocturnal light should be a high priority in the hospital environment. Both Pisani and Hardin address nocturnal light levels and note that levels above 100 lux have been shown to affect melatonin secretion, while levels above 300 lux may affect the circadian pacemaker. Lighting levels in the ICU can often exceed 1000 lux, and nocturnal use can have a significant impact on sleep disruption. Impaired sleep and circadian disruption is a well-known cause of delirium in the hospital setting and may place patients at risk. Patients, particularly the elderly, who experience episodes of delirium while in the hospital may have poorer outcomes and have a documented increase in 6–12 month mortality in multiple studies [3–5].

  Light is not the only factor affecting sleep in the hospital. Patient surveys post-hospitalization show that noise and talking are frequently reported disruptive activities affecting sleep, although PSG data within this environment reveals that only 10–30% of arousals are due to noise [1]. Despite attempts to facilitate an environment that is quiet and restful, daily hospital activities can contribute to significant noise pollution. Daytime noise levels often range from 55 to 65 dB, and peak noise levels above 80 dB are associated with arousals from sleep. The EPA recommends that noise levels remain below 40 dB during the day and below

35 dB at night. There is additional evidence to suggest that abrupt changes in noise levels may be more disruptive than overall decibel peaks. A study that evaluated the effect of continuous low-level background white noise exposure within the ICU may support this assertion and demonstrated a reduction in noise-related arousals [6]. Attempts should be made to limit unnecessary noise by turning off televisions and phones when not in use and during the night. Staff and visitors should avoid conversations at the bedside when patients are resting. Consideration should be given to instituting limits on the number of visitors at the bedside and require visitors to adhere to posted visiting hours.

Patient monitoring activities, especially the acquisition of vital signs, are reported by patients to be the most disruptive to sleep in the hospital [1]. Patients are often attached to three or more monitoring devices (EKG, pulse-ox, BP, etc.) while inpatient to help facilitate their care. These devices often have both visible lights and audible noise associated with their routine functioning. Additionally, these cables may restrict mobility and cause irritation and sleep disruption. Others may be more invasive, like automated blood pressure cuffs, and directly stimulate the patient, which can increase arousals. Patient monitors should be kept on privacy settings to limit lights, and noise and automated monitoring devices should be set for the longest appropriate interval with monitoring done from a central location.

Direct patient care actives can be very disruptive to sleep. Some of these care activities include scheduled medication administration, bathing and wound care, diagnostic imaging (i.e., bedside and overnight studies, MRI, CT), procedures, and lab testing (i.e., line placement, catheter placement, blood draws). Studies have shown that patients can have an average of 40–60 direct patient contacts overnight for these types of activities [1, 2].

Approximately 10% of patient awakenings during 24 hours are due to patient care activities [1]. Nightly care activities (bathing, meds) should be coordinated and performed early in the evening before lights out. Attempts should be made to maintain a sleep hygiene protocol (door closed, lights out, curtains closed, television off) during the night to minimize patient disruptions. Nighttime studies and procedures should be deferred to daytime hours unless urgent or emergent need arises. Often despite efforts to minimize interruptions and awakenings, patients will still struggle to sleep during the night. Up to 50% of total sleep time (TST) in the ICU is "made up for" during the daytime hours [1]. Allowance of extended daytime sleep periods should be considered on an individual patient basis as this may significantly decrease the homeostatic sleep drive and potentially result in nocturnal insomnia and further circadian dysrhythmia.

- *The patient is sedated, but does that mean they are resting and getting adequate sleep?*

  It is essential to recognize that sedation does not equate to sleep, and many of the sedative and analgesic medications used in the ICU affect sleep. In a 2009 review article on sleep in the ICU, Hardin provided a review of the effects of many common ICU sedatives and medication affecting sleep. One of the commonly used classes of sedative agents used in the ICU is anxiolytic agents (i.e., benzodiazepines [BZD]). BZDs activate GABA-A receptors and affect norepinephrine (NE) and glutamate secretion. This class of medication has been shown at low doses to decrease sleep latency (SL), increase total sleep time (TST), decrease spindle activity, decrease slow-wave sleep (SWS), and increase cortical arousals. High doses suppress cerebral function causing diffuse slowing (delta waves) with decreased EEG amplitude. BZD in the ICU setting is typically used for specific processes (like alcohol or BZD withdrawal and seizure) or short-term procedural sedation due to their high risk for potentiating delirium.

Propofol, a novel general anesthetic that is frequently used in the ICU, is thought to act on GABA-A and NMDA receptors, and its effects on sleep are similar to those of the BZD class [1]. In a small study of 40 ICU patients, Treggiari-Venzi assessed the effect of overnight sedation with midazolam versus propofol on sleep quality as well as depression and anxiety scores. The study demonstrated comparable outcomes on the quality of sleep and reestablishment of circadian rhythm without improvement of anxiety or depression [7 (PMID 9120111)].

Another commonly used sedative agent, dexmedetomidine (DEX), is a novel alpha-2 receptor agonist that induces sedation and decreases agitation but allows natural arousal and causes little respiratory suppression. Infusions produce a state similar to stage N2 sleep, though with an overall decrease in the total amount of time in stage R [8, 9]. Several studies are evaluating the effect of DEX on sleep in critically ill patients. DEX has been suggested to decrease the incidence of delirium, agitation, and confusion in critically ill patients in a meta-analysis of 3029 patients [10 (PMID 25034724)]. In a small pilot study of 13 ICU patients who were hemodynamically stable and ventilated in an assist control or spontaneous ventilation mode, DEX infusion overnight to a RASS −1 to −2 improved sleep efficiency and decreased sleep fragmentation while shifting to a more standard 24-hour sleep pattern [11]. Additional more extensive powered studies are needed to verify these findings, but this pilot study does suggest that DEX may be useful in maintaining a more standardized sleep pattern in selected stable ICU patients.

Ketamine, a non-competitive NMDA receptor antagonist, is another sedative that is sometimes used in the ICU. Ketamine has multiple beneficial effects in critically ill patients to include sedation, analgesic, hypnotic, and amnestic effects. It also has the benefit of a minimal impact on respiratory drive and has been shown to activate the upper airway muscles and preserve pharyngeal and laryngeal reflexes [12]. There are multiple studies evaluating ketamine's effects on sleep in various patient populations. One small case-control study examined its effects in the critically ill by looking at 40 burn patients who received ketamine infusion with overnight PSG and comparing them to 20 matched controls to determine the effects on sleep. The significant impact on sleep architecture was an overall reduction in stage R, but a similar effect was seen in the control group who did not receive ketamine. Interestingly, ketamine administration did not affect nocturnal TST, several awakenings, time awake after sleep onset, and the percent of time spent in stage N1, N2, or N3(+4) [13]. Findings from this limited study suggest that ketamine may be useful for sedation with a less significant impact on sleep architecture compared to other sedative agents.

• *There are many known classes of medications that affect the sleep cycle through modulation of CNS receptors or their neurotransmitters. What are some of the commonly used medications in the ICU that have effects on both peripheral and central nervous systems that affect sleep, and how can I limit their impact on my patient's sleep cycle?*

Frequently, medications used in the ICU are specifically chosen for their effects on the CNS in an attempt to control pain, reduce agitation, stabilize mood, or prevent seizures. Many peripherally acting medications used to stabilize blood pressure and cardiac function or improve pulmonary function also have possible secondary effects on the CNS. Other medications that work to modulate or boost the immune system or decrease inflammation may also impact sleep by modulating neurotransmitters and suppressing melatonin secretion.

Pain management is a frequent issue during critical illness or injury. Ensuring adequate analgesia may have significant effects on a patient's ability to participate in rehabilitation, their mood and affect, and their ability to obtain adequate sleep. Opiate medications are frequently used for their pain modulating and sedating effects on the mu receptors throughout the nervous system. Non-steroid anti-inflammatory drugs (NSAID) are also often employed to assist in reducing the number of opiates a patient receives while helping to ease pain and inflammation by suppressing prostaglandin synthesis. Both opiates and NSAIDs are often sedating and decrease TST, SWS, REM, and sleep efficiency (SE) [1].

Several classes of soporific medications have been evaluated within the hospital setting. Melatonin has been evaluated in several small studies within the ICU. The effects of critical illness on the pattern of melatonin secretion are mixed and conflicting with data suggesting both increases and decreases in endogenous secretion with various degrees of illness and the use of invasive mechanical ventilation [14]. Within the existing literature, studies evaluating the effects of exogenous melatonin administration have likewise been conflicting. One study looking at ICU patients with chronic obstructive pulmonary disease (COPD) demonstrated improved TST and sleep quality with a 3 mg dose of melatonin nightly [14]. A separate study of mechanically ventilated patients receiving 10 mg melatonin during their weaning period also showed a similar benefit [14]. Conversely, a study of critically ill patients with tracheostomy demonstrated no difference in subjectively assessed sleep parameters following the administration of 3 mg melatonin [14].

Interestingly, melatonin may exert some effect on the level of analgesia needed in the ICU. In a 2015 RCT study of 1158 ICU patients by Mistraletti, administration of 3 mg melatonin at 8 PM and midnight showed a decrease in the number of sedative agents required and appeared to improve pain, agitation, and anxiety [15]. Several prospective studies are currently underway to further clarify the role of melatonin in the management of critically ill patients and the prevention of delirium. A more recent alternative to exogenous melatonin administration that has been evaluated in the ICU is direct melatonin receptor agonists such as ramelteon. While no inpatient studies have addressed its potential soporific effects, ramelteon was shown in a study of 67 elderly patients (age 65–89) to decrease the incidence of delirium when compared to placebo [16].

Sedative hypnotic medications, such as the non-benzodiazepine receptor agonists (e.g., zolpidem and eszopiclone), have also been evaluated for use within the hospital environment. In the outpatient setting, these medications have been demonstrated to improve several sleep-related parameters. However, within the inpatient setting, studies have suggested increasing incidences of delirium, falls, and cognitive dysfunction, particularly in the elderly [17–20]. For these reasons, sedative-hypnotics should be utilized with caution, if not avoided, within the intensive care unit, particularly in elderly patients and those at risk for delirium.

Anti-anxiolytic (i.e., benzodiazepines) agents may be used for anxiety and sedation in the ICU, as previously discussed. This class of medicine works via the stimulation of GABA receptors and may have some effect on endocannabinoid receptors. They are sedating and increase TST and stage N2 sleep, though they have also been observed to decrease REM and SWS duration [1]. Tricyclic anti-depressants (TCA) are sometimes used as sleep aids or for depression in the ICU. They function by stimulating alpha-1 receptors and suppressing muscarinic activity. This class of medicine may be sedating and increase TST and stage N2 sleep while suppressing stage R [1]. Selective serotonin reuptake inhibitors (SSRI) and selective norepinephrine reuptake inhibitors (SNRI) have also been used in the ICU to help with depression, especially during prolonged ICU admissions. Both classes increase 5-HT (5-hydroxytryptamine, aka serotonin) activity, with SNRIs having secondary effects increasing NE activity. Both classes tend to increase TST and decrease SWS, REM, and SE [1].

Anti-epileptic drugs (AED) are often used in the ICU to halt and suppress seizure activity. Many works by affecting sodium channels in the CNS through GABA and glutamate receptors, which suppress cell depolarization. This frequently causes significant sedation along with an increase in TST. Additionally, they will result in decreased SL and often cause suppression of SWS [1]. Dopamine agonists used for the treatment of Parkinson's disease are also often seen in the elderly ICU patient population. These tend to be sedating and cause a reduction in SWS, along with an increased incidence of nightmares [1].

Many patients in the ICU require some level of cardiovascular support, and many have underlying cardiovascular disease processes, which are more challenging to control when critically ill. Atrial fibrillation with the rapid ventricular response is commonly seen in ICU patients and is often managed with beta-blockers (BB) for rate control. In addition to the targeted cardiovascular beta receptors, there is also secondary CNS blockade, which may affect sleep. Within the CNS, BB may be activating, thereby causing more frequent awakenings while suppressing REM and increasing the incidence of nightmares [1]. Hypotension is also frequently encountered in ICU patients, and the use of peripherally acting vasoactive stimulant medications that target alpha, beta, and dopamine receptors is common. Most of these agents also work on receptors in the CNS, causing activation and suppression of REM and SWS [1].

Antihistamines may be used during acute drug reactions or anaphylaxis episodes to help stabilize airway swelling. They are also often employed for their antiemetic effects and sedating properties. Interacting with the H1 histamine receptor and affecting acetylcholine secretion, they may induce significant sedation. Corticosteroids are also frequently used to decrease inflammation and suppress immune function. Systemic corticosteroids have long been known to cause sleep disturbance, often decreasing stage R and SWS and occasionally inducing nightmares [1].

- *When a patient is on a noninvasive ventilator, how can I optimize ventilator settings to maximize sleep quality and efficiency?*

Patients frequently arrive at the emergency department in acute distress after struggling with an illness, which affected their quality and quantity of sleep for hours to days. When a patient arrives in respiratory distress, they may be placed on NIPPV in an attempt to stabilize and temporize them until additional testing or procedures can be performed. In a patient who does not have altered mentation and can protect their airway, NIPPV can be an effective way to support respiration. Patients will not infrequently require extended time on NIPPV and will typically sleep while on this mode of ventilation. Patient synchrony with the ventilator can often be one of the most significant factors affecting sleep.

The goal of NIPPV is to improve ventilation and gas exchange, and offload a portion of the work of the inspiratory muscles while decreasing the overall work of breathing. To achieve this effect, continuous positive airway pressure (CPAP) or bilevel positive airway pressure ventilation (BPAP) is often used to reduce the effort needed during inspiration and help prevent airway and alveolar collapse during expiration.

Bilevel ventilation with an inspiratory pressure setting (IPS) and end-expiratory pressure (EEP) that targets a driving pressure or tidal swing of 40–80% is effective in gas exchange, which improves sleep efficiency and percent of the time in stage R in chronically ventilated patients with neuromuscular disease [21]. Reasonable initiation pressures for NIPPV have been evaluated in stable COPD patients. An average IPS of 15+/−3 cm H_2O and EEP of 3.1+/−1.6 cm H_2O was effective in improving ABG values and unloading the work of breathing [22]. These initial pressures should be adjusted based on the individual mechanics of the patient to provide maximal support and benefit.

- *My patient has failed NIPPV or arrived in respiratory failure and was intubated and is currently on invasive ventilation. How can I optimize their ventilator setting to improve sleep?*

Mechanically ventilated patients in the ICU experience a poor quality of sleep. In these patients, polysomnographic studies have demonstrated increased sleep fragmentation, a reduction in slow-wave (stage N3) sleep and stage R sleep, as well as an abnormal distribution of sleep [23]. Prior studies have attributed environmental noise and patient care activities to about 30% of arousals and awakenings in mechanically ventilated patients in the ICU; however, the etiology of the triggering factors for the remainder of the sleep fragmentation is unclear

[24, 25]. Mechanical ventilation has been investigated for its role as a direct mechanism for sleep disruption. Potential variables of mechanical ventilation that may contribute to sleep disruption include mode of ventilation, improper ventilator settings, and patient-ventilator asynchrony [1].

Several small studies have evaluated the direct effect of mechanical ventilation modes in relation to sleep quality in critically ill patients. One small randomized crossover study of 11 sedated critically ill patients observed an increase in central sleep apneas (CSA) and sleep fragmentation when the ventilatory mode was switched from assist-control ventilation (ACV) to pressure support ventilation (PSV) without a backup rate. It is unclear whether the PSV mode itself or the potential excess ventilatory support was the cause of the CSAs; however, it is worth noting that five of the six patients who developed CSAs had a history of congestive heart failure [26], which may have been an independent risk factor. In a cross-over study of 35 non-sedated patients on mechanical ventilation, pressure control ventilation (PCV) resulted in improved sleep quality and quantity compared to low-level PSV (low-PSV) defined as 6 cm H_2O [27]. When ACV mode was compared to low-PSV in a randomized cross-over study of 20 non-sedated patients weaning from mechanical ventilation, there was significantly improved sleep architecture with ACV mode. However, when Cabello compared automatically adjusted PSV to clinician-adjusted PSV and ACV in 15 non-sedated patients, there was no difference in sleep between the groups [23]. Compared to spontaneous breathing, PSV was only associated with better sleep quantity but not quality in non-sedated difficult-to-wean patients with tracheostomies [28].

The mode of mechanical ventilation during sleep may not be as important as the role of patient ventilatory effort. In a study of ambulatory ventilated patients with neuromuscular disease, an improvement in sleep quality, specifically, sleep architecture and nighttime gas exchange, was observed when the pressure support (PS) level was adjusted to match the patients' respiratory effort during sleep and wakefulness [21]. As demonstrated by Cabello, sleep improved when the patient's effort was synchronous with PSV settings, likely due to decreased requirements for pressure support and positive end-expiratory pressure [23]. When proportional assist ventilation (PAV) was compared with PSV in 13 sedated patients, PAV was found to be more efficacious than PSV in matching ventilatory requirements [29]. The improved patient-ventilator synchrony likely resulted in improved sleep architecture due to fewer arousals and awakenings.

While specific ventilator modes demonstrated improved sleep quality in certain small studies, this finding is likely explained by decreased patient-ventilator asynchrony and reduction of ineffective efforts. In order to reduce sleep disruptions in ICU patients on mechanical ventilation, the focus should be on instituting a comprehensive ventilator strategy rather than a specific mode or settings that matches ventilator assistance with the patient's ventilatory requirements and underlying pulmonary mechanics. Large randomized studies are still required to compare specific ventilator modes, settings, and variables of patient-ventilator interactions.

- *During illness, the body responds by increasing inflammation through the release of cytokines and chemokines to help assist with recovery; how are these factors affecting my patient's sleep and should I attempt to modulate their effects?*

The majority of cytokine and chemokines, when evaluated in animal models, have been shown to increase NREM, with the exceptions being IL-4, IL-10, and IL-13, all which had the opposite effect of decreasing NREM sleep [2, 30]. IL-1, IL-6, tumor necrosis factor (TNF), and interferon (INF) have all been more extensively evaluated in regard to their effects during illness.

IL-1 and TNF are key factors in the inflammatory cascade activated during infection and have been shown to affect GABA and serotonergic systems in both healthy and ill individuals. When one or both is elevated, they may cause stage R suppression and increased SWS activity and NREM sleep [30]. IL-6 is an important downstream mediator of IL-1 and TNF response. Elevated levels of IL-6 in animal models have been shown to affect sleep during states of immune response by suppressing stage R and increasing SWS and NREM [30]. IL-6 levels have also been shown to be elevated in patients with health conditions that cause excessive daytime sleepiness and in persons who are deprived of sleep [30].

There has been less research on the effects of INF on sleep; however, data from animal studies show that elevated levels are associated with increased NREM and a reduction in REM latency. Sleep disruptions in patients with viral infections suggest that INF likely has a similar effect in humans [30].

In the ICU setting, patients with overwhelming infection and injury can frequently have an excessive and hyper-exaggerated cytokine response, which may lead to secondary physiologic insults and clinical instability. Many of the interventions that are made are intended to stabilize and support the patient while the body has time to mount an effective response to illness. The effects of impaired and lost sleep on recovery and overall outcome during critical illness are not known at this time, but some animal studies show that increases in SWS and NREM are associated with better outcomes [30]. If the animal models are reflective of the same processes within humans, it would suggest that promoting NREM sleep could improve outcomes in critically ill patients.

General Remarks

Sleep disturbances frequently occur in critically ill patients in the ICU and have been linked to the development of delirium, prolonged stay in the ICU, and increased mortality [3]. There are numerous factors, both modifiable and non-modifiable, that contribute to sleep impairment in the ICU. Our patient has a high risk for sleep impairment due to his admission to the ICU, critical illness, and required treatment modalities. While certain environmental factors can be modified, like light, noise, and unnecessary patient care interruptions at night, patient-specific factors like pain control, anxiety, and preexisting sleep disorders should be assessed routinely for optimization. As several common medications have been shown to affect sleep quality and architecture negatively, the provider must remain attentive to the iatrogenic effects of prescribed medications on sleep quality [2]. In mechanically ventilated patients, patient-ventilator synchrony is an essential factor for sleep quality and quantity. The relationship between severity of illness and sleep disturbances in the ICU environment is complicated. In our patient with septic shock and respiratory failure requiring mechanical ventilation and sedative medications, the pathophysiology of his inflammatory condition and required treatment modalities contribute to his sleep fragmentation. Ultimately, sleep deprivation in critically ill patients must be recognized as preventable harm, and a multifaceted approach must be instituted to address modifiable risk factors.

Pearls/Take Home Points
- Recognize that all critically ill patients are at high risk for sleep disturbances due to a variety of modifiable and non-modifiable factors.
- Adequate pain control and limitation of patient-care activities during typical sleeping hours are likely the two most important modifiable factors for decreasing sleep disturbances in ICU patients.
- Many commonly used sedative and analgesic medications negatively affect the quality of sleep in critically ill patients.
- Providers must routinely review an ICU patient's medication list to avoid unnecessary negative iatrogenic effects on sleep quality.
- In mechanically ventilated patients, patient-ventilator synchrony is the most important factor for sleep quality and quantity.

References

1. Hardin KA. Sleep in the ICU. Chest. 2009;136(1):284–94. https://doi.org/10.1378/chest.08-1546.
2. Pisani MA, Friese RS, Gehlbach BK, Schwab RJ, Weinhouse GL, Jones SF. Sleep in the intensive care unit. Am J Respir Crit Care Med. 2015:731–738. https://doi.org/10.1164/rccm.201411-2099CI.
3. Ely EW. Delirium as a predictor of mortality in mechanically ventilated patients in the intensive care unit. JAMA. 2004;291(14):1753. https://doi.org/10.1001/jama.291.14.1753.
4. Mccusker J, Cole M, Abrahamowicz M, Primeau F, Belzile E. Delirium predicts 12-month mortality. Arch Intern Med. 2002;162(4):457. https://doi.org/10.1001/archinte.162.4.457.
5. Leslie DL, Zhang Y, Holford TR, Bogardus ST, Leo-Summers LS, Inouye SK. Premature death associated with delirium at 1-year follow-up. Arch Intern Med. 2005;165(14):1657. https://doi.org/10.1001/archinte.165.14.1657.
6. Stanchina ML, Abu-Hijleh M, Chaudhry BK, Carlisle CC, Millman RP. The influence of white noise on sleep in subjects exposed to ICU noise. Sleep Med. 2005;6(5):423–8. https://doi.org/10.1016/j.sleep.2004.12.004.
7. Treggiari-Venzi M, Borgeat A, Fuchs-Buder T, Gachoud J-P, Suter PM. Overnight sedation with midazolam or propofol in the ICU: effects on sleep quality, anxiety, and depression. Intensive Care Med. 1996;22(11):1186–90. https://doi.org/10.1007/bf01709334.

8. Mason KP, O'Mahony E, Zurakowski D, Libenson MH. Effects of dexmedetomidine sedation on the EEG in children. Pediatr Anesth. 2009;19(12):1175–83. https://doi.org/10.1111/j.1460-9592.2009.03160.x.

9. Huupponen E, Maksimow A, Lapinlampi P, et al. Electroencephalogram spindle activity during dexmedetomidine sedation and physiological sleep. Acta Anaesthesiol Scand. 2008;52(2):289–94. https://doi.org/10.1111/j.1399-6576.2007.01537.x.

10. Pasin L, Landoni G, Nardelli P, et al. Dexmedetomidine reduces the risk of delirium, agitation, and confusion in critically ill patients: a meta-analysis of randomized controlled trials. J Cardiothorac Vasc Anesth. 2014;28(6):1459–66. https://doi.org/10.1053/j.jvca.2014.03.010.

11. Alexopoulou C, Kondili E, Diamantaki E, et al. Effects of dexmedetomidine on sleep quality in critically ill patients. Anesthesiology. 2014;121(4):801–7. https://doi.org/10.1097/aln.0000000000000361.

12. Canet J, Castillo J. Ketamine. Anesthesiology. 2012;116(1):6–8. https://doi.org/10.1097/aln.0b013e31823da398.

13. Gottschlich MM, Mayes T, Khoury J, Mccall J, Simakajornboon N, Kagan RJ. The effect of ketamine administration on nocturnal sleep architecture. J Burn Care Res. 2011;32(5):535–40. https://doi.org/10.1097/bcr.0b013e31822ac7d1.

14. Boyko Y, Jennum P, Toft P. Sleep quality and circadian rhythm disruption in the intensive care unit: a review. Nat Sci Sleep. 2017;9:277–84. https://doi.org/10.2147/nss.s151525.

15. Mistraletti G, Umbrello M, Miori S, et al. Melatonin reduces the need for sedation in ICU patients: a randomized controlled trial. Minerva Anestesiol. 2015;81(12):1298–310.

16. Hatta K, Kishi Y, Wada K. Ramelteon for delirium in hospitalized patients. JAMA. 2015;314(10):1071. https://doi.org/10.1001/jama.2015.8522.

17. Mahoney JE, Webb MJ, Gray SL. Zolpidem prescribing and adverse drug reactions in hospitalized general medicine patients at a Veterans Affairs Hospital. Am J Geriatr Pharmacother. 2004;2(1):66–74.

18. Richards K, Rowlands A. The impact of zolpidem on the mental status of hospitalized patients older than age 50. Medsurg Nurs. 2013;22(3):187–91.

19. Mangusan RF, Hooper V, Denslow SA, Travis L. Outcomes associated with postoperative delirium after cardiac surgery. Am J Crit Care. 2015;24(2):156–63.

20. Kolla BP, Lovely JK, Mansukhani MP, Morgenthaler TI. Zolpidem is independently associated with an increased risk of inpatient falls. J Hosp Med. 2013;8(1):1.

21. Fanfulla F, Delmastro M, Berardinelli A, Lupo ND, Nava S. Effects of different ventilator settings on sleep and inspiratory effort in patients with neuromuscular disease. Am J Respir Crit Care Med. 2005;172(5):619–24. https://doi.org/10.1164/rccm.200406-694oc.

22. Vitacca M, Nava S, Confalonieri M, et al. The appropriate setting of noninvasive pressure support ventilation in stable COPD patients. Chest. 2000;118(5):1286–93. https://doi.org/10.1378/chest.118.5.1286.

23. Cabello B, Thille AW, Drouot X, et al. Sleep quality in mechanically ventilated patients: comparison of three ventilatory modes. Crit Care Med. 2008;36(6):1749–55. https://doi.org/10.1097/ccm.0b013e3181743f41.

24. Freedman NES, Gazendam J, Levan L, Pack AI, Schwab RJ. Abnormal sleep/wake cycles and the effect of environmental noise on sleep disruption in the intensive care unit. Am J Respir Crit Care Med. 2001;163(2):451–7. https://doi.org/10.1164/ajrccm.163.2.9912128.

25. Gabor JY, Cooper AB, Crombach SA, et al. Contribution of the intensive care unit environment to sleep disruption in mechanically ventilated patients and healthy subjects. Am J Respir Crit Care Med. 2003;167(5):708–15. https://doi.org/10.1164/rccm.2201090.

26. Parthasarathy S, Tobin MJ. Effect of ventilator mode on sleep quality in critically ill patients. Am J Respir Crit Care Med. 2002;166(11):1423–9. https://doi.org/10.1164/rccm.200209-999oc.

27. Andréjak C, Monconduit J, Rose D, et al. Does using pressure-controlled ventilation to rest respiratory muscles improve sleep in ICU patients? Respir Med. 2013;107(4):534–41. https://doi.org/10.1016/j.rmed.2012.12.012.

28. Roche-Campo F, Thille AW, Drouot X, et al. Comparison of sleep quality with mechanical versus spontaneous ventilation during weaning of critically ill tracheostomized patients. Crit Care Med. 2013;41(7):1637–44. https://doi.org/10.1097/ccm.0b013e318287f569.
29. Bosma K, Ferreyra G, Ambrogio C, et al. Patient-ventilator interaction and sleep in mechanically ventilated patients: pressure support versus proportional assist ventilation. Crit Care Med. 2007;35(4):1048–54. https://doi.org/10.1097/01.ccm.0000260055.64235.7c.
30. Opp MR. Cytokines, and sleep. Sleep Med Rev. 2005;9(5):355–64. https://doi.org/10.1016/j.smrv.2005.01.002.

Part VII

Other Sleep and Co-morbid Issues

Nocturnal Panic Disorder: Afraid to Sleep!

15

Vijaya Bharathi Ekambaram, Irina Baranskaya,
and Britta Klara Ostermeyer

Clinical Case History

Mrs. Smith is a 33-year-old married, unemployed, mother of three young children, who presented as a new patient to establish outpatient psychiatric services. She reports experiencing severe stress recently. She has been experiencing significant marital issues and suspects that her husband is unfaithful. Her husband lost his job recently, and they are experiencing significant financial struggles. In addition, her 5-year-old son has difficulties adjusting to kindergarten.

Mrs. Smith has a prior history of depression and anxiety disorder and previously saw a psychiatrist several years ago who prescribed some medication that she cannot recall. For the past two years, she has been unable to follow-up with any doctors due to lack of insurance.

Also, Mrs. Smith reports a trauma history: During her college years, her ex-boyfriend choked and attempted to rape her but she was able to escape. Mrs. Smith has a long-standing history of daytime panic attacks. She describes these episodes as intense fear of dying accompanied by palpitations, sweating, shortness of breath, choking sensations, and dizziness. She states that these daytime panic attacks are usually triggered by being in crowded places. She avoids going out shopping in anticipated fear of these panic attacks.

Mrs. Smith reports worsening of her panic disorder for the past month. She states that she began having panic attacks at night at least once a week. She reports waking up at night with intense fear of dying followed by chest discomfort, palpitations,

V. B. Ekambaram
Touro University California, Vallejo, California, USA

I. Baranskaya · B. K. Ostermeyer (✉)
University of Oklahoma Health Sciences Center, Department of Psychiatry and Behavioral Sciences, Oklahoma City, OK, USA
e-mail: britta-ostermeyer@ouhsc.edu

© Springer Nature Switzerland AG 2021
I. S. Khawaja, T. D. Hurwitz (eds.), *Sleep Disorders in Selected Psychiatric Settings*, https://doi.org/10.1007/978-3-030-59309-4_15

gasping for air, and choking sensations. She reports waking up rather abruptly prior to a nocturnal panic attack without any triggers or nightmares. These attacks usually last less than 10 minutes, and she is unable to fall back to sleep after these nocturnal awakenings. Mrs. Smith's typical bedtime is 11:00 pm and these nocturnal panic attack episodes usually occur around 1:00 am. While she reports no issues in falling asleep, she stresses that lately she is afraid to go to sleep due to her nocturnal panic attacks.

Physical Examination and Mental Status Examination

Mrs. Smith is 65 inches (165 cm) tall and weighs 138 lbs (63 kg). Her BMI is with 23.1 in the normal range, and her vital signs are normal as well. She is a well-nourished female, neatly groomed and dressed, and looking her stated age. She is cooperative and forthcoming with the examination. She exhibits no abnormal movements, and her gait is normal. Her speech is normal. She describes her mood as "so stressed out and exhausted due to family issues and lack of sleep," and her affect is anxious. Her thought processes are normal, and she states no perceptual abnormalities and no suicidal or homicidal ideations. She is oriented to person, date, time, place, and situation, and her cognition is intact. She is able to name recent events in popular media, was able to do serial 7-s correctly, and her abstract thinking is intact as well.

Results

Mrs. Smith's blood counts, thyroid stimulating hormone (TSH), and blood chemistries were within normal limits. Her urine drug screen (UDS) was negative. Brain CT scan, EEG, and EKG were unremarkable as well.

Mrs. Smith underwent a diagnostic polysomnography (PSG), and the results were within normal limits. There were no snoring or obstructive events noted. EEG montage did not detect any epileptiform activity. There were no periodic limb movements or complex behaviors or parasomnias documented either, and her sleep stage architecture was normal as well.

Differential Diagnosis

Mrs. Smith's abrupt nocturnal awakening can be caused by multiple conditions, including nocturnal panic disorder, sleep terrors, post-traumatic stress disorder (PTSD), sleep paralysis, sleep apnea, nocturnal epilepsy, and/or medication withdrawal. Considering this larger differential diagnosis, we should consider the following:

Table 15.1 Main features of nocturnal panic attacks

Usually occurring in adults
No obvious trigger
Abrupt awakening from sleep within the first 1–3 hours of sleep onset
More somatic and respiratory symptoms
Reduction in heart period variability
Difficulties falling back to sleep
Eventually development of fear association with sleep by patient
Association with autonomic dysfunction and increase in sympathetic activation
Occurs in NREM sleep particularly during transition from stage II to stage III without any electroencephalographic abnormalities
All laboratory and test workup may be normal

1. Nocturnal panic disorder (NPD) is defined as abrupt arousal from sleep with a sense of fear, palpitations, shortness of breath, chest discomfort, feelings of unreality, choking sensation, and hot or cold flashes [1]. NPD's presentation, quality, and duration may appear similar to daytime panic disorder but NPD occurs without any obvious trigger or environmental stimuli (see Table 15.1). The attacks typically happen between 1 and 3 hours after sleep onset, last between 2 and 8 minutes, and usually occur once per night. Patients typically complain about difficulties in returning to sleep and are usually able to recall these attacks later on [2]. Mrs. Smith, who has a history of daytime panic disorder, started to develop nocturnal panic as her predominant symptom. In Mrs. Smith's case, NPD occurred within 3 hours of sleep onset, lasted less than 10 minutes, and occurred without any obvious triggers. She also reported difficulties falling back to sleep and was able to recall the attacks later on.

2. In contrast to NPD, sleep terrors predominantly occur during slow-wave sleep (stage IV sleep) with abrupt awakenings usually in childhood and adolescence. Patients cry and scream, are able to return back to sleep rather quickly, and do not recall the event, with caregivers usually reporting these incidents. Mrs. Smith has no childhood history of night terrors, sleepwalking, or parasomnias, and she is clearly able to remember these nocturnal episodes.

3. Nightmares in patients with PTSD occur during REM sleep typically in the latter half of the night. These nocturnal awakenings are primarily triggered by trauma-related events and images. In Mrs. Smith's case, these episodes usually happened in the first half (within 3 hours of sleep onset) of the night during non-REM sleep and occurred abruptly without trauma reminders or triggers.

4. Sleep paralysis and sleep-related hallucinations occur because of dysfunctional overlap between REM sleep and wakefulness. Patients experience it when they are about to fall asleep or about to wake up from sleep and are unable to speak and unable to perform voluntary movements. They also have hallucinatory experiences and fears and are fully able to recall these vivid dream experiences and images. These events frequently occur in individuals with narcolepsy. Mrs. Smith has no movement paralysis and no hallucinatory experiences.

5. Some seizure types, such as juvenile myoclonic and awakening grand mal, benign Rolandic, electrical status epilepticus of sleep, and Landau-Kleffner syndrome (LKS), have strong predilection toward sleep. These nocturnal seizures are usually associated with EEG abnormalities. Mrs. Smith had a normal EEG, which clearly rules out nocturnal seizure disorder.

6. Sleep apnea is usually triggered by risk factors, such as obesity and crowded airways. Patients with sleep apnea present with symptoms of snoring, gasping for air, frequent awakenings, and daytime sleepiness. Sleep apnea patients' PSG clearly document repeated obstructive events and respiratory cessation throughout the night from stages I, II, and REM sleep. In NPD patients, nocturnal awakening followed by respiratory cessation is typically a single time occurrence without frequent repetitions [2, 3]. Mrs. Smith has no sleep apnea risk factors or symptoms, and her PSG did not document any obstructive events.

7. Sometimes nocturnal awakenings can also be triggered by withdrawals from medications, such as benzodiazepines [2]. Mrs. Smith has no history of benzodiazepine use and her urine drug screen was negative.

Final Diagnosis

Mrs. Smith's history, examination, laboratory findings, and sleep study are compatible with nocturnal panic disorder (NPD), which is a subtype of panic disorder.

Discussion

Nocturnal panic disorder (NPD) is considered as a distinct subgroup of panic disorder and about 70% of panic disorder patients experience NPD at some point in their lifetime (Need ref. here). Despite this high life-time prevalence, only 45% of panic disorder patients have recurrent history of NPD [4]. While there are significant overlaps between nocturnal and diurnal panic attacks in their presentation, their etiology and underlying mechanism remain unclear. Despite these overlaps, there are key features which differentiate nocturnal from diurnal attacks (see Table 15.1).

Compared to daytime panic attacks, nocturnal panic attacks abruptly emerge without any triggers, such as agoraphobia or situational and environmental factors [2, 5]. However, patients with NPD eventually often develop fearful associations with sleep and sleep-like states, such as meditation and relaxation [5]. Researchers have found elevated emotional reactivity to conditions resembling sleep state in NPD and have suggested that fear of loss of vigilance and reduction in awareness could be contributing to developing fearful associations with sleep in NPD [2]. These fearful sleep associations eventually cause patients to avoid going to sleep and lead to sleep onset delays and chronic sleep deprivations [2].

NPD patients typically experience more somatic sensations and more frequent respiratory symptoms (shortness of breath, gasping for air, choking) compared to patients with daytime panic attacks [6]. Some biological models hypothesized that respiratory symptoms in NPD are due to respiratory dysregulations such as carbon dioxide receptor hypersensitivity and chronic hyperventilation. However, these studies lack empirical support and further research is warranted to confirm this hypothesis [7].

In a study investigating ambulatory sleep heart period variability (HPV) among groups of patients with NPD and daytime panic attacks and groups of non-anxious patients, the results showed that NPD patients have significant reduction in HPV compared to daytime panic attack patients and non-anxious patients [8]. The authors hypothesized that reduction in HPV and faster heart rate in NPD individuals were possibly related to a lack of vagal tone which in turn triggered an increased sympathetic activity [8]. Cardiac presentation is one of the main precipitants for NPD, with a prior diagnosis of mitral valve prolapse found in a higher proportion of patients with NPD. Further investigations are needed to explore the role of cardiac symptoms in NPD [2].

Whereas few studies reported that daytime panic attacks are driven primarily by cognitive and psychological factors, NPD is influenced more by biological factors, such as autonomic nervous system dysfunction and increases in sympathetic activation [6].

Increased bodily movements have been documented during sleep in patients with panic disorder compared to controls, and these increased sleep-related movements are considered to be a protective factor against NPD [7]. Some biological models hypothesized that reduced movement time during sleep combined with heightened vulnerability to relaxation form the underlying pathogenesis of NPD [7]. However, further studies are warranted to confirm these findings.

Frequent awakenings, non-restorative sleep, chronic sleep deprivation, and insomnia are frequent complaints of patients with NPD [9], and impaired arousal regulation was found to be the underlying cause for these NPD-related sleep problems [9]. Objective evidence was found in polysomnographic studies, which have documented decreases in sleep efficiency and sleep duration in patients with panic disorder [1, 9].

Depression can also cause sleep disturbances, including problems in sleep onset with shortened REM latency, sleep maintenance, early morning awakenings, and excessive daytime sleepiness [1, 9]. NPD and depression are independently and interactively associated with sleep disturbances, and 92.3% of patients reported sleep disturbances when they had both depression and NPD [1].

While few researchers have documented that patients with NPD have more severe anxiety, are more prone to suicidality, and have higher incidences of comorbid depression, childhood history of anxiety, and sleep disturbances compared to diurnal panic attacks, these findings were not repeated in other studies [4].

Detailed sleep assessment and mental health assessment are needed to confirm NPD diagnosis and to rule out other conditions, such as depression, anxiety, PTSD, sleep terrors, sleep paralysis, sleep apnea, and nocturnal epilepsy. Information about patients' current and past sleep habits and daily monitoring of sleep-related behaviors are essential in arriving at a diagnosis, and the Stanford sleepiness scale as well as daily sleep logs can be helpful during the evaluation [2]. Mental health assessment using semi-structured diagnostic interviews can assist in diagnosing or ruling out anxiety disorders, mood disorders, PTSD, and other substance use related disorders. Tools such as Anxiety Disorders Interview Schedule-IV (ADIS-IV) and Structured Clinical Interview for DSM (SCID) can be used for screening anxiety disorders, mood disorders, somatoform disorders, psychosis, and substance-related disorders.

The Nocturnal Panic Screen Scale developed by Craske and colleagues in 2005 is a valuable NPD screening tool, helping to gather detailed information about frequency, time of onset, behavioral changes, and anticipatory sleep anxiety associated with NPD [2]. Polysomnography is not routinely performed for diagnosing NPD. Typically, NPD occurs in non-rapid eye movement (NREM) sleep, particularly during transition from stage II to stage III without any electroencephalographic abnormalities. While studies have found an increase in sleep latency, decreased sleep time, decreased sleep efficiency, and less slow wave sleep in polysomnography in patients with NPD, these studies were limited by sample size, by lack of an adaptation night, and by medication influences [2]. In clinical practice, sleep polysomnography and upper air way resistance measurements (esophageal pressure monitoring) are usually performed to rule out other sleep disorders such as sleep apnea. In recent years, ambulatory monitoring devices have been utilized in some studies to capture physiology associated with NPD. In contrast to single night polysomnography, these devices can record and provide more physiological information continuously for prolonged intervals up to 60 hours [2, 10].

Regarding treatment of NPD, pharmacological approaches are limited due to lack of randomized control trials. Some case reports and case series have shown that alprazolam (dosing up to 5 mg) and tricyclic antidepressants to be effective in NPD cessation [2, 11].

Cognitive behavior therapy (CBT) for NPD has shown significant reduction in NPD symptom severity and frequency, and treatment effects can last up to 2 years following treatment [2, 12, 13]. CBT sessions (usually 11 sessions, each of 60 minutes in duration) target both daytime and nighttime panic attacks. Initial sessions provide patients with education about the physiological anxiety process and about how heightened sensitivity to sensations of anxiety causes fluctuations in sleep physiology. Fear can cause arousals followed by nocturnal panic attacks [2, 12]. The CBT technique of cognitive restructuring addresses the misappraisals of bodily sensations and catastrophizing associated with dysfunctional beliefs, and breathing retraining in CBT can be used as a coping skill to overcome shortness of breath and choking during nocturnal episodes. CBT also educates patients about basic sleep hygiene measures and how to improve poor sleep habits [2, 12, 13].

Outcome of Case

Mrs. Smith underwent a detailed mental health and sleep assessment and was diagnosed with depressive disorder, anxiety disorder, and NPD. She was started on fluoxetine for anxiety and was enrolled in CBT to target her symptoms of depression, anxiety, and NPD. She underwent a total of 12 weekly CBT sessions. Her progress was monitored by using sleep logs and the Nocturnal Panic Screen Scale. At the end of her CBT sessions, she reported marked reduction in her NPD symptoms and frequency.

Take Home Points
- Nocturnal panic disorder (NPD) is a distinct subgroup of panic disorder typically occurring in adult patients who wake up abruptly usually during in the first 1–3 hours after sleep onset. Patients wake up in a state of panic without any obvious triggers and usually experience more somatic and respiratory symptoms. They have difficulties falling back to sleep and recall the episode later on.
- NPD has more underlying biological mechanisms, such as autonomic nervous system dysfunction and an increase in sympathetic activation, compared to diurnal panic attacks which are usually driven by underlying cognitive and psychological factors.
- Patients with NPD require thorough mental health and sleep assessment. Laboratory workup and tests such as a polysomnography might be normal.
- CBT has shown promising progress in the treatment of NPD.

References

1. Singareddy R, Uhde TW. Nocturnal sleep panic and depression: relationship to subjective sleep in panic disorder. J Affect Disord. 2009;112(1–3):262–6. https://doi.org/10.1016/j.jad.2008.04.026. Epub 2008 Jun 16. PMID: 18558437.
2. Craske MG, Tsao JC. Assessment and treatment of nocturnal panic attacks. Sleep Med Rev. 2005;9(3):173–84. Epub 2005 Apr 8. Review. PubMed PMID: 15893248.
3. Craske MG, Lang AJ, Mystkowski JL, Zucker BG, Bystritsky A, Yan-Go F. Does nocturnal panic represent a more severe form of panic disorder? J Nerv Ment Dis. 2002;190(9):611–8. PubMed PMID: 12357095.
4. Norton GR, Norton PJ, Walker JR, Cox BJ, Stein MB. A comparison of people with and without nocturnal panic attacks. J Behav Ther Exp Psychiatry. 1999;30(1):37–44. PubMed PMID:10365864.
5. Sarísoy G, Böke O, Arík AC, Sahin AR. Panic disorder with nocturnal panic attacks: symptoms and comorbidities. Eur Psychiatry. 2008;23(3):195–200. Epub 2007 Oct 15. PubMed PMID: 17937981.
6. Shapiro CM, Sloan EP. Nocturnal panic--an underrecognized entity. J Psychosom Res. 1998;44(1):21–3. PubMed PMID: 9483461.

7. Craske MG, Lang AJ, Rowe M, DeCola JP, Simmons J, Mann C, Yan-Go F, Bystritsky A. Presleep attributions about arousal during sleep: nocturnal panic. J Abnorm Psychol. 2002;111(1):53–62. PubMed PMID: 11866179.

8. Aikins DE, Craske MG. Sleep-based heart period variability in panic disorder with and without nocturnal panic attacks. J Anxiety Disord. 2008;22(3):453–63. Epub 2007 Mar 18. PubMed PMID: 17449220.

9. Overbeek T, van Diest R, Schruers K, Kruizinga F, Griez E. Sleep complaints in panic disorder patients. J Nerv Ment Dis. 2005;193(7):488–93. PubMed PMID: 15985844.

10. King RJ, Bayon EP, Clark DB, Taylor CB. Tonic arousal and activity: relationships to personality and personality disorder traits in panic patients. Psychiatry Res. 1988;25:65–72.

11. Mellman TA, Uhde TW. Patients with frequent sleep panic: clinical findings and response to medication treatment. J Clin Psychiatry. 1990;51:513–6.

12. Barlow DH, Gorman JM, Shear MK, Woods SW. Cognitive behavioral therapy, imipramine, or their combination for panic disorder: a randomized controlled trial. JAMA. 2000;283(19):2529–36.

13. Craske MG, Brown TA, Barlow DH. Behavioral treatment of panic disorder: a two-year follow-up. Behav Ther. 1991;22:289–304.

Psychosocial Issues of Narcolepsy

16

Neelam Danish, Ani Gupta, Ayesha Ebrahim, Omo Edaki, and Imran S. Khawaja

Clinical History

A 31-year-old married Caucasian male, a resident in radiology (Dr. X), came to the sleep center, referred by his psychiatrist for concerns of not being able to stay asleep at night.

Dr. X had been seeing a psychiatrist as he has been under immense stress at work and has been treated for depression and anxiety. As a resident in radiology, he has to be on call multiple times during the week and has to be in a dark room when reading radiographs and other tests. Being in a dark room makes it very difficult for Mr. X to stay awake, and he falls asleep while reading the X-rays or CT scans. At times his fellow trainees make jokes about him, which resulted in some interpersonal friction among the colleagues. He is falling behind on his reports and gets phone calls from his supervisors who have complained to his residency training director.

He has trouble getting to work on time as he often cannot wake up on alarms. Excessive daytime sleepiness has got worse since he started his second year of residency. His residency training director has given him warnings and put him on probation as he has been late for morning conferences consistently.

N. Danish
Cardiovascular Surgery, UT Southwestern Medical Center, Dallas, TX, USA

A. Gupta
The Ohio State Wexner Medical Center, Department of Neurology, Columbus, OH, USA

A. Ebrahim
Endocrinology, MD TruCare, Grapevine, TX, USA

O. Edaki
Department of Psychiatry Clinical Research, John Peter Smith Hospital, Fort Worth, TX, USA

I. S. Khawaja (✉)
MD TruCare PA, Grapevine, TX, USA

Department of Psychiatry, The University of Oklahoma, OK, USA

© Springer Nature Switzerland AG 2021
I. S. Khawaja, T. D. Hurwitz (eds.), *Sleep Disorders in Selected Psychiatric Settings*, https://doi.org/10.1007/978-3-030-59309-4_16

He is getting more irritable at home as he worries about his career and finishing his residency. Even at home, he tries to remote into work so he could catch up on the unfinished reports. His wife is unhappy as she feels that he does not give time to her and their 4-year-old daughter. His wife (also a resident in Internal Medicine) feels he is not helping in the household work, which has caused even more resentment in her.

On weekends, when he is not working, he tries to spend time with the family, but often sleeps during the daytime. He does not feel like going out, which makes his wife unhappy, and they now have been getting into arguments frequently. He has not been able to visit his family and friends even on holidays as he tries to catch up on his work.

He has always been a "sleepyhead" even in medical school but somehow managed using high amounts of caffeinated beverages. He has attributed his sleepiness to not getting enough sleep, but now it is affecting his functioning at work and home. He is becoming isolated socially and is having problems in his married life. He is getting more depressed and is worrying about his career. Other residents try not to bother him as he is irritable and gets upset quickly.

The patient's wife reports that he falls asleep minutes after watching TV or reading a book. He wakes up four to five times at night, each episode characterized by difficulty returning to sleep. He attributes his awakenings to nightmares and, at times, not being able to move his body during these episodes.

He denies any restless legs symptoms or abnormal breathing events during sleep. During the daytime, he uncontrollably and abruptly finds himself falling asleep for short durations. He denies any falls from the sudden loss of muscle tone.

His psychiatrist had prescribed amitriptyline 150 mg for depression, anxiety, and sleep fragmentation, but it has worsened daytime sleepiness. The patient started psychotherapy for his anxiety once a week, but more recently, the worsening of his daytime sleepiness has caused him to miss several appointments.

Particularly worrisome to him is an increased propensity of falling asleep while driving.

His past medical, surgical, and psychiatric histories are unremarkable, except for depression and anxiety. His family history is significant for bipolar disorder and insomnia in his mother. The patient denies any use of illicit drugs or stimulants.

Diagnostic Evaluation

On physical examination, Mr. X appears to be well groomed, in no apparent distress but appears to be tired. He is mildly obese with a BMI of 30 and a neck size of 16.5 inches. His neurological examination is unremarkable. He scores 21/52 points on the Hamilton Depression Rating Scale, indicating severe depression. His Epworth Sleepiness Scale score is 19.

The sleep physician ordered both a polysomnogram (PSG) and the Multiple Sleep Latency Test (MSLT). Total sleep time of 7 hours 55 minutes demonstrated a significantly reduced REM latency of 10 minutes and multiple spontaneous awakenings with an arousal index of 15 per hour. His sleep efficiency was low (78%), and there was an increase in his stage N1 and N2 sleep. Notably, no apneic phases, snoring, choking, or periodic limb movements were present during his sleep study.

His MSLT captured five nap sections. Mean sleep latency was 6 minutes, with 3 Sleep Onset REM Periods (SOREMS).

Mr. X's clinical presentation and results from the PSG, MSLT were highly suggestive of narcolepsy. Cerebrospinal fluid (CSF) analysis of orexin-A/hypocretin-1 showed 40 pg/ml, which was highly suggestive of narcolepsy type 1.

Questions

Can a person have narcolepsy without any symptoms of cataplexy? What are the most common psychosocial problems associated with narcolepsy? Does the treatment of narcolepsy improve comorbid conditions such as depression and anxiety?

Differential Diagnosis

1. Idiopathic Hypersomnia

    Idiopathic hypersomnia is characterized by the absence of cataplexy and hypocretin-1 deficiency (which distinguishes it from narcolepsy). Diagnosis requires an MSLT showing a mean sleep latency of <8 minutes with fewer than two sleep-onset REM periods (SOREMPs) [1]. Furthermore, there is an increase in total sleep time, sleep efficiency, and deep NREM sleep, as well as short sleep latencies. Contrary to narcolepsy, these patients complain of un-refreshing long naps and difficulty arousing from sleep.

2. Kleine-Levin Syndrome

    Kleine-Levin syndrome (aka sleeping beauty syndrome) is characterized by recurrent episodes of severe hypersomnia associated with cognitive and behavioral disturbances. Episodes may last for days to weeks. There is an increase in total sleep time often more than 18 hours/day with typical sleep structure, mild reduction in sleep efficiency due to frequent awakenings during NREM stages N1 & N2, and a reduced time spent in N3 stages.

3. Neurological Disorders

    Excessive daytime sleepiness (EDS) can present in illnesses that adversely affect the cerebral cortex bilaterally or deep midline structures that are critical for maintaining alertness.

4. Medical conditions/Medications

    Metabolic/endocrine disorders have been associated with EDS as having a variety of medications such as benzodiazepine, non-benzodiazepine sedatives, antihistamine, anticonvulsants, opioids, sedating antidepressants, and antipsychotics.

General Remarks

Dr. X's clinical presentation and diagnostic workup are consistent with the diagnosis of "narcolepsy type 1," even though he did not have cataplexy as his hypocretin levels were low. Narcolepsy is a chronic sleep disorder with abnormal regulation of sleep/wake cycles that are characterized by excessive daytime sleepiness (EDS) as well as cataplexy. Dr. X did not have cataplexy which refers to sudden, transient episodes of loss of muscle tone without loss of consciousness, which occur in response to intense emotions (i.e., laughter, anger, surprise, or humor). It is often associated with fragmented nighttime sleep and hypnopompic and hypnagogic hallucinations. Low levels of hypocretin 1/orexin A (less than 110 pg/ml) in the cerebrospinal fluid are highly specific for narcolepsy type 1.

According to the International Classification of Sleep Disorders (ICSD)-3, narcolepsy type 1 is defined as excessive daytime sleepiness (EDS) and at least one of the following criteria: (a) cataplexy and a positive MSLT or (b) hypocretin deficiency. An MSLT is considered positive when the mean sleep latency is ≤8 minutes and when there are two or more sleep-onset REM periods (SOREMPs). Hypocretin deficiency is defined as cerebrospinal fluid (CSF) hypocretin 1 level < 1/3 of normal or ≤ 110 pg/ml.

Pathogenesis of narcolepsy involves the destruction of hypocretin-producing cells of the ventral hypothalamus in genetically susceptible individuals that are carriers of one or more alleles of HLA DQB1*0602 locus, possibly by autoimmune processes as evidenced by T-cell polymorphism, infections (i.e., streptococcus and H1N1 influenza), and H1N1 vaccination.

Psychosocial Issues of Narcolepsy

Patients with narcolepsy suffer challenges in everyday life. These include difficulties with social relationships, poor academic performances, occupational maladjustments, increased health care expenses, and risk of accidents. These factors may contribute to worsening underlying psychiatric comorbidities.

Narcoleptic patients are often labeled as "lazy" by their family members and teachers. They have trouble maintaining alertness, which affects their performance in school and at work. Excessive daytime sleepiness poses great difficulty in maintaining their relationships and socialization. There is a lack of public understanding of this disorder and its potential therapy. Patients are often viewed as being lazy, which may lead to negative attitudes and additional emotional pressures, as well as to challenges in marital, work, and interpersonal relationships. Therefore, educational interventions aimed at increasing awareness and encouraging social interactions, support groups, and interventions, family counseling, structured, regular activities, and self-monitoring of symptoms could improve academic, neurobehavioral, and psychosocial functioning.

Patients who develop narcolepsy in childhood may also suffer a decline in academic performances. "Mental fog," difficulty thinking, remembering, concentrating, and paying attention are the most commonly reported symptoms. Children are often misdiagnosed as having ADHD, or in cases of narcolepsy with atypical cataplexy (that is atypical due to static appearance or dyskinetic movements), they are misdiagnosed as having epilepsy. Misdiagnosis inadvertently leads to delayed treatment. Early recognition and correct diagnosis would help in preventing or slowing of academic decline.

Many narcoleptics such as Mr. X are unable to keep up with their work schedules, especially if they have to do shift work, and many of these patients ultimately go on full disability. According to a study done by Naumann [2], narcoleptics suffer from deficits in attention and all executive functions, whereas memory and routine alertness tasks are either unaffected or only mildly impaired. Despite the sound quality of performance, reduced capacity to maintain a sufficient level of alertness for more extended periods and decline in information processing compromise occupational performance, which over some time leads to professional incompatibility.

Psychiatric disorders are common in adults with narcolepsy. Patients with narcolepsy have increased rates of depression (24.8%) and anxiety (17.7%) [3]; although the exact cause of depression is not known, an increase in daytime sleepiness along with disturbed nighttime sleep has been shown to lead to depression [3]. Also, it has been shown that a decrease in hypocretin levels is associated with amygdala dysfunction. It is hypothesized that the changes in affective modulation in the amygdaloidal neural system could lead to pathological emotional processes, which ultimately could result in major depression.

Patients with narcolepsy are continually at risk of motor vehicle accidents due to sleep attacks, as reported in several studies (for patients with idiopathic hypersomnia and narcolepsy). According to one study [4] by Ozaki et al., 55% of current narcoleptic drivers had at least one automobile accident or near-miss incident within the past 5 years. Some states have regulations against patients with narcoleptic individuals to have a commercial driver's license. Needless to say that patients with narcolepsy cannot be airplane pilots.

Narcolepsy is associated with a significant socioeconomic burden due to both high direct and indirect health care costs. Early disease onset, lack of curative treatment, the need for life-long symptomatic treatment as well as reduced functioning of the patient with a significant portion of narcoleptics becoming functionally disabled are major contributing factors. The annual direct medical cost is estimated to be twice as high as compared to matched individuals without narcolepsy ($11,702 vs. $5261, $p < 0.0001$) [5].

According to Black et al. [6], narcoleptics had higher annual rates of inpatient admissions and outpatient visits as compared to controls. Comparison of ratios in narcoleptics and controls showed twofold higher rates in inpatient admissions (0.15 vs. 0.08), emergency department (ED) visits w/o admission (0.34 vs. 0.17), hospital outpatient (OP) visits (2.8 vs. 1.4), other OP services (7.0 vs. 3.2), and physician visits (11.1 vs. 5.6), all ratios with a $p < 0.0001$. The rate of total annual drug transactions was twice as high in narcoleptic patients versus controls (26.4 vs. 13.3; $p < 0.0001$). Mean yearly costs were significantly higher in narcoleptic patients compared to controls for medical services ($8346 vs. $4147; $p < 0.0001$) and prescription medications ($3356 vs. $1114; $p < 0.0001$).

Management

In the case of Dr. X, the sleep physician wrote a letter to the training director to minimize on-call work, which significantly helped with daytime sleepiness. Mr. X was also started on sodium oxabate at night and methylphenidate during the daytime, which improved his alertness to a point where he was no more dozing off at work and was able to focus and complete his work. His performance improved over the next few months, and he was taken off probation. Daytime alertness improved his social and interpersonal life. The wife commented, "I wish he would have been prescribed these medications ten years ago." The sleep doctor educated the wife about the disorder and also suggested that Dr. X takes a nap of a few minutes even on the weekends, which further improved alertness.

Impaired quality of life and social dysfunction are significant complaints of patients with narcolepsy. Behavioral measures, such as scheduled naps, improved sleep hygiene, and diet control, play a significant role in ameliorating symptoms [7]. Sleep physicians recommend daily naps at work as these measures can improve the quality of work and reduce occupational stress.

Cognitive-behavioral therapy for narcolepsy (CBT-N), which includes a (i) behavioral component that focuses on sleep satiation and nap training and a (ii) cognitive component that aims at modifying beliefs, emotions, and motivation, has been shown to improve psychosocial issues associated with narcolepsy [8]. Patient education can help raise awareness about strategies in dealing with the socioeconomic aspects of the disease. Systematic desensitization and lucid dreaming have been shown to help with cataplexy and hallucinations, respectively.

Pharmacotherapy controls the symptoms and helps patients in better adapting to the psychosocial problems referred to above. Modafinil and other stimulants (armodafinil, amphetamine, methamphetamine, dextroamphetamine, methylphenidate) are effective in treating narcolepsy. Selective serotonin reuptake inhibitors (SSRI), tricyclic antidepressants (TCA), and venlafaxine have been used to treat cataplexy. Sodium oxybate is useful for narcolepsy with cataplexy. At a dose of 4.5 g twice nightly, it has been shown to alleviate all of the symptoms of narcolepsy with cataplexy. However, its use is strictly regulated in both the USA and Europe due to its potential for abuse (mind-altering agent).

> **Clinical Pearls**
>
> The clinicians should address psychiatric, economic, and social comorbidities in addition to medical management in order to provide more comprehensive and effective treatment for patients with narcolepsy.
>
> Behavioral therapy and social support, along with pharmacological treatment, can play a significant role in relieving the psychosocial burden of narcolepsy.

References (Suggested Reading)

1. American Academy of Sleep Medicine. International classification of sleep disorders. 3rd ed. Darien: American Academy of Sleep Medicine; 2014.
2. Naumann A, Bellebaum C, Daum I. Cognitive deficits in narcolepsy. Journal of sleep research. J Sleep Res. 2006;15:329–38.
3. Maski K, Steinhart E, Williams D, et al. Listening to the patient voice in narcolepsy: diagnostic delay, disease burden, and treatment efficacy. J Clin Sleep Med. 2017;13(3):419–25.
4. Akiko Ozaki RN, Inoue Y, Nakajima T. Health-related quality of life among drug-naïve patients with narcolepsy with cataplexy, narcolepsy without cataplexy, and idiopathic hypersomnia without long sleep time. J Clin Sleep Med. 2008;4(6):572–8.
5. Thorpy MJ, Hiller G. The medical and economic burden of narcolepsy: implications for managed care. Am Health Drug Benefits. 2017;10(5):233–41.
6. Black J, Reaven NL, Funk SE, et al. The Burden of Narcolepsy Disease (BOND) study: healthcare utilization and cost findings. Sleep Med. 2014, 15: 522-529.
7. Kapella MC, Berger BE, Vern BA, et al. Health-related stigma as a determinant of functioning in young adults with narcolepsy. PLoS One. 2015;10(4):e0122478.
8. Agudelo HAM, Correa UJ, Sierra JC, Pandi-Perumal SR, Schenck CH. Cognitive-behavioral treatment for narcolepsy: can it complement pharmacotherapy? Sleep Sci. 2014;7(1):30–42.

Severe OSA and Claustrophobia, Ultimately Treated with Hypoglossal Nerve Stimulation

17

Bibi Aneesah Jaumally, Teresa Chan-Leveno, and Won Young Lee

Clinical History/Case

Ms. E is a 67-year-old morbidly obese female with severe depression and refractory anxiety referred to sleep clinic for management of severe obstructive sleep apnea (OSA). OSA had been diagnosed years prior, but she was intolerant to continuous positive airway pressure (CPAP) due to intense claustrophobia associated with vivid visual hallucinations. She had an extreme phobia about pests and CPAP markedly exacerbated this phobia to the point of uncontrollable tears. Moreover, she was fearful about being "anchored" to a CPAP device which could prevent her escape from bed should rodents infest her bed. Multiple attempts were made to acclimate to CPAP including (1) desensitization sessions, (2) initiation of sleep hypnotic agents, (3) cognitive behavioral therapy, and (4) optimization of her treatment of anxiety and depression, all of which were unsuccessful. The phobia evolved to intense emotional outbursts even at the very sight of the machine.

Due to the concerns that untreated OSA was exacerbating her mood disorder, alternatives to CPAP were sought including referral for a mandibular advancement device, which was unsuccessful. She also underwent bariatric surgery, and despite significant weight loss, her repeat polysomnogram again revealed severe OSA.

Finally after continued concerns that untreated severe OSA and sleep fragmentation were exacerbating her psychiatric disorders, she was considered for

B. A. Jaumally
UT Health Science Center at Houston, Department of Internal Medicine, Houston, TX, USA

T. Chan-Leveno
University of Texas Southwestern Medical Center, Department of Otolaryngology, Dallas, TX, USA

W. Y. Lee (✉)
University of Texas Southwestern Medical Center, Department of Internal Medicine, Dallas, TX, USA
e-mail: Won.Lee@utsouthwestern.edu

© Springer Nature Switzerland AG 2021
I. S. Khawaja, T. D. Hurwitz (eds.), *Sleep Disorders in Selected Psychiatric Settings*, https://doi.org/10.1007/978-3-030-59309-4_17

hypoglossal nerve stimulation (HGNS) therapy. She underwent careful evaluation between sleep medicine, psychiatry, and otolaryngology before moving forward with surgical implantation of the hypoglossal nerve stimulator. A repeat polysomnogram performed after surgical implantation of the stimulator revealed successful treatment of obstructive sleep apnea and hypoxemia. She endorsed improved quality of sleep and better control of depression on antidepressants.

Examination/Mental Status Exam

On initial examination, she was tearful throughout the interview and her affect was severely depressed. Her Epworth Sleepiness Scale was 15/24. Her vital signs were within normal limits. Cardiopulmonary and neurological examinations were also normal.

Results

Diagnostic polysomnography revealed an apnea-hypopnea index (AHI) of 21 with a nadir oxygen saturation of 72%. Repeat polysomnography after bariatric surgery and weight loss redemonstrated severe OSA with an AHI of 39 and nadir oxygen saturation of 72% (Fig. 17.1a, b). Her HGNS post-activation polysomnogram study revealed markedly improved AHI of only 4.6 events per hour at the optimal amplitude of 1.8 volts with nearly complete resolution of associated hypoxemia (Fig. 17.2a, b).

Questions

1. Does treatment of comorbid OSA improve intractable depression?
2. What are the treatment options available for patients with OSA and claustrophobia?

Differential Diagnosis and Diagnosis

The patient has severe OSA and intolerance to CPAP due to intense claustrophobia.

General Remarks

There is a higher prevalence of depression in patients with OSA than the general population, and symptoms of depression and untreated OSA may often overlap [1, 2]. Untreated OSA can be associated with antidepressant treatment failure [2]. Sleep fragmentation and hypoxemia in OSA may lead to depression. Moreover, low levels

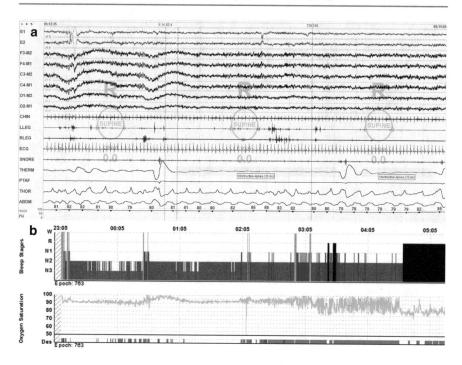

Figs. 17.1 (**a, b**) Diagnostic polysomnography: 90-second epochs depicting obstructive apneas in supine REM and hypnogram with significant oxygen desaturations

of serotonin seen in depression may lead to development of OSA by decreasing serotonin delivery to the dilator pharyngeal muscles which in turn have a higher tendency to collapse during sleep [1]. There is evidence that treatment of OSA may lead to improved mood, decreased depression and anxiety, as well as an overall improvement in psychological health and quality of life [2]. Further, the treatment of OSA can also lead to improved compliance to pharmacological treatment for depression and may lead to better clinical response to antidepressants. Significant decreases in depression symptoms and anxiety have been seen in patients with OSA treated with CPAP and with oral surgery. On the other hand, treatment of concomitant depression has been hypothesized to improve adherence and acceptance of OSA therapy [2].

More than 60% of patients with OSA complain of claustrophobic tendencies related with CPAP. This is more common in women and can lead to poor adherence to CPAP. CPAP desensitization, changing to a different interface namely nasal mask or nasal pillows instead of a full face mask, cognitive behavioral therapy, mandibular advancement device, and weight loss are acceptable treatment options and alternatives. HGNS is a novel and effective treatment approach for patients with moderate to severe OSA who have not tolerated first-line therapies [3]. Relevant to our case, HGNS has been successfully used to treat OSA and has been found to substantially decrease symptoms of depression as well as improve quality of life measures up to 1 year post-implantation.

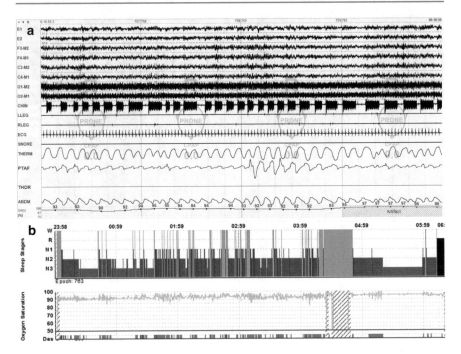

Figs. 17.2 (**a**, **b**) HGNS treatment polysomnography – 2-minute epoch depicting REM in the prone position with successful treatment of obstructive apneas and hypnogram with improved sleep quality and improved oxygen saturations

---

Pearls/Take Home Points

1. Depression and OSA present with overlapping symptoms and often coexist in clinical practice. Diagnosis and treatment of OSA should be considered in depressed patients to improve the likelihood of successful treatment of depression.

2. In patients with OSA who are unable to tolerate PAP therapy despite desensitization and who have a history of depression, oral appliances or HGNS should be considered to improve OSA and alleviate OSA-related symptoms, in addition to improving recalcitrant depression.

References

1. Ejaz SM, Khawaja IS, Bhatia S, Hurwitz TD. Obstructive sleep apnea and depression. Innov Clin Neurosci. 2011;8(8):17–25.
2. Schroder CM, O'Hara R. Depression and obstructive sleep apnea. Ann Gen Psychiatry. 2005;4:13.
3. Strollo PJ, Soose RJ, Maurer JT, de Vries N, Cornelius J, Froymmovich O, et al. Upper-airway stimulation for obstructive sleep apnea. N Engl J Med. 2014;370(2):139–49.

Neuropsychological Outcomes of Disordered Sleep

18

Case Study: Obstructive Sleep Apnea. "I'm Forgetting Conversations"

Christopher T. Copeland, Jessica Holster, and Morgan B. Glusman

Clinical History/Case

Mr. C is a 55-year-old Caucasian man with hypertension, hyperlipidemia, hypercholesterolemia, recurrent major depressive disorder, and untreated obstructive sleep apnea (OSA). He was referred by his primary care physician for a neuropsychological evaluation of his cognitive complaints. On initial interview, he complained of excessive daytime sleepiness, intermittent memory loss, word-finding difficulty, distractibility, increased irritability, and trouble staying asleep at night of approximately 4 years' duration. He denied problems with expressive or receptive language, problem solving, or abstract thinking. He denied anhedonia, persistent sadness, worry, or a history of alcohol or illicit substance use. He denied problems with instrumental activities of daily living or activities of daily living.

Social History

Mr. C lives with his wife. He is employed as a high school math teacher. He earned a bachelor's degree in education. He reported earning mostly A's and B's throughout school. His favorite and least favorite academic subjects throughout school were math and English, respectively. He denied a history of learning problems or special education classes throughout school. He denied work performance problems aside from occasionally forgetting some of his students' names and sporadically losing track of his thoughts during classroom lectures.

C. T. Copeland (✉) · J. Holster · M. B. Glusman
The University of Oklahoma, College of Medicine, Department of Psychiatry & Behavioral Sciences, Neuropsychology Lab, Oklahoma City, OK, USA
e-mail: christopher-copeland@ouhsc.edu

© Springer Nature Switzerland AG 2021
I. S. Khawaja, T. D. Hurwitz (eds.), *Sleep Disorders in Selected Psychiatric Settings*, https://doi.org/10.1007/978-3-030-59309-4_18

Evaluation Methods

Prior to beginning continuous positive airway pressure (CPAP) treatment, Mr. C participated in an initial neuropsychological evaluation. He returned for a repeat neuropsychological evaluation following 12 consecutive months of nightly CPAP treatment. During both appointments, he was administered tests designed to measure several different aspects of his cognitive functioning. Three comparison standards were utilized to assess cognitive functioning. First, Mr. C's test scores were compared to test scores produced by demographically matched peers. Second, Mr. C's test scores were compared to his estimated premorbid functioning. Third, Mr. C's pre- and post-CPAP test scores were compared to help determine if his cognitive functioning improved following CPAP treatment. Improved cognitive test performance following CPAP treatment would suggest the presence of transient cognitive inefficiencies associated with sleep disruption prior to CPAP treatment. Stable or worsening cognition following CPAP treatment may suggest possible vascular cognitive impairment and/or another neurocognitive disorder.

Clinical Observations

Mr. C was timely; casually dressed and appropriately groomed; alert; oriented to the current date, month, year, day, place, and city; and polite and cooperative during both of his appointments. His thoughts were linear and goal directed. He frequently yawned and complained of fatigue throughout his initial evaluation. He appeared well-rested during his second evaluation. He adequately engaged in the testing process.

Evaluation 1 Test Results

Attention span, information processing speed, and memory recall were excessively variable across similar tests administered throughout the evaluation. Attention span was worse on repetitive tasks and better on intellectually stimulating tasks. Alternating attention and response inhibition were mildly impaired. Visuospatial functioning, memory recognition, language, abstract thinking, and intellectual functioning were consistently above average on all tests administered throughout the day. Mood screeners suggested mild depression and did not suggest anxiety.

Evaluation 2 Test Results

Test performances were less variable during Mr. C's second evaluation. Overall, he performed above average on most tests of attention span, information processing speed, visuoconstruction, language, memory recall, memory recognition, abstract thinking, and intellectual functioning. Mood screeners did not suggest depression or anxiety.

Question

What aspect of sleep disturbance best explains Mr. C's cognitive inefficiencies during his initial evaluation?

Diagnostic Impressions

During his first evaluation, Mr. C's excessively variable attention, information processing speed, and memory recall with otherwise broadly intact cognitive functioning were consistent with impaired vigilance and sleep disruption. Improvement in these cognitive domains following CPAP compliance for 12 months further supported impressions of transient cognitive inefficiencies.

General Remarks

Disturbed sleep is associated with impaired cognitive and daily functioning. The duration and nature of cognitive deficits are influenced by disordered sleep duration, sleep fragmentation, sleep variability, circadian time synchronization, excessive daytime sleepiness, and/or associated physiologic changes [1]. Routine cognitive assessments help detect cognitive deficits as well as predict and measure response to treatment over time. Further evaluation of emotional and behavioral symptoms that may present with disrupted sleep (i.e., health problems, emotional changes, behavioral problems) is also important.

Sleep Duration

Chronic, long sleep duration (often defined as ≥9 nightly hours) is associated with impaired attention and information processing speed in older adults [2, 3] and impaired general cognition, memory, and mental flexibility in middle-aged adults [4] and has predicted 1-year incident amnestic cognitive impairment in older men [5]. Chronic, short sleep duration (often defined as ≤5 or ≤6 nightly hours) is associated with impaired attention and information processing speed in older adults [2, 3] and with decreased memory, visuomotor speed, and reaction time in adolescents with a greater impact on women's reaction time [6, 7]. Transient sleep loss is often associated with little to no consequence on cognition among healthy adults and may be as or less impactful on cognitive test performances than the impact of pain, medication side effects, age, and years of education [8]. In children, chronic sleep loss may be associated with lower full scale IQ and verbal IQ [9] and with subtle inefficiencies in executive functioning, school performance, and performance on tasks that are reliant on integration of multiple skills [7, 9].

Sleep Fragmentation

Sleep fragmentation in some older adult samples has been associated with incident dementia and an over 20% increase in the annual rate of cognitive decline at 6-year follow-up [10]. Sleep fragmentation due to compromised rapid eye movement (REM) sleep mechanisms is a prominent feature of narcolepsy. Despite memory complaints in up to nearly half of patients with narcolepsy, these patients' memory test performances are often normal [11]. Memory loss complaints among patients with narcolepsy may be best explained by deficits in attention [12], decreased vigilance on repetitive and uninteresting but not novel tasks [13], depression [14], or anxiety [15]. Sleep fragmentation due to frequent awakenings is a well-documented aspect of SAS. Sleep fragmentation in SAS samples has been associated with variable vigilance and potentially reversible deficits in attention, information processing speed, verbal fluency, manual dexterity, and memory [16–18]. CPAP treatment may improve verbal learning capability in as little as two nights [18] and manual dexterity, memory, and information processing speed within 3 months [16]. OSA may impact children's attention/concentration, executive functioning, visual-motor and spatial skills, nonverbal reasoning, memory, and motor dexterity [19–22]. Inefficiencies in these areas may resolve with tonsillectomy and adenotonsillectomy [22–24]. Hyperactivity in response to sleep loss is a unique feature in children that contributes to sleep fragmentation [24, 25].

Physiologic Changes

Physiologic changes associated with some sleep disorders may lead to irreversible cognitive deficits. Cerebrovascular changes due to severe nocturnal hypoxemia in SAS may lead to enduring deficits in intelligence and executive functioning [16–18, 26]. Idiopathic REM sleep behavior disorder is associated with a substantially increased risk for synucleinopathic neurodegenerative diseases such as multiple system atrophy, dementia with Lewy bodies, and Parkinson's disease [27]. Chronic sleep loss may lead to loss of white matter integrity [28], and only one night of sleep loss may lead to transiently increased levels of a protein in Alzheimer's pathology (Aβ42) [29]. The influence of chronic and severe sleep disruption during early brain development is unclear and complex but may exert a long-standing, cumulative effect on brain structure and function [30], body composition, emotion regulation, growth, and blood pressure [25, 30].

Pearls/Take-Home Points
Transient sleep disruption is associated with subtle and transient cognitive inefficiencies in attention, information processing speed, and lower-order executive functioning. Chronic sleep disruption associated with some sleep disorders may lead to enduring physiologic changes, cognitive deficits, and an increased risk for a neurodegenerative disorder.

References

1. Kelly DA, Coppel DB. Sleep disorders. In: Tarter RE, Butters M, Beers SR, editors. Medical neuropsychology. 2nd ed. New York: Kluwer Academic/Plenum Publishers; 2001. p. 267–84.
2. Blackwell T, Yaffe K, Ancoli-Israel S, Redline S, Ensrud KE, Stefanick ML, Laffan A, Stone KL. Associations between sleep architecture and sleep-disordered breathing and cognition in older community-dwelling men: the Osteoporotic Fractures in Men Sleep Study. J Am Geriatr Soc. 2011;59(12):2217–25. https://doi.org/10.1111/j.1532-5415.2011.03731.x.
3. Blackwell T, Yaffe K, Ancoli-Israel S, Redline S, Ensrud KE, Stefanick ML, Laffan A, Stone KL. Association of sleep characteristics and cognition in older community-dwelling men: the MrOS sleep study. Sleep. 2011;34(10):1347–56. https://doi.org/10.5665/sleep.1276.
4. van Oostrom SH, Nooyens ACJ, van Boxtel MPJ, Verschuren WMM. Long sleep duration is associated with lower cognitive function among middle-age adults - the Doetinchem Cohort Study. Sleep Med. 2018;41:78–85. https://doi.org/10.1016/j.sleep.2017.07.029.
5. Potvin O, Lorrain D, Forget H, Dube M, Grenier S, Preville M, Hudon C. Sleep quality and 1-year incident cognitive impairment in community-dwelling older adults. Sleep. 2012;35(4):491–9. https://doi.org/10.5665/sleep.1732.
6. Sufrinko A, Johnson EW, Henry LC. The influence of sleep duration and sleep-related symptoms on baseline neurocognitive performance among male and female high school athletes. Neuropsychology. 2016;30(4):484–91. https://doi.org/10.1037/neu0000250.
7. Short MA, Blunden S, Rigney G, Matricciani L, Coussens S, M Reynolds C, Galland B. Cognition and objectively measured sleep duration in children: a systematic review and meta-analysis. Sleep Health. 2018;4(3):292–3000. https://doi.org/10.1016/j.sleh.2018.02.004.
8. Seelye A, Mattek N, Howieson D, Riley T, Wild K, Kaye J. The impact of sleep on neuropsychological performance in cognitively intact older adults using a novel in-home sensor-based sleep assessment approach. Clin Neuropsychol. 2015;29(1):53–66. https://doi.org/10.1080/13854046.2015.1005139.
9. Astill RG, Van der Heijden KB, Van Ijzendoom MH, Van Someren EJ. Sleep, cognition, and behavioral problems in school-age children: a century of research meta-analyzed. Psychol Bull. 2012;138(6):1109–38. https://doi.org/10.1037/a0028204.
10. Lim AS, Kowgier M, Yu L, Buchman AS, Bennett DA. Sleep fragmentation and the risk of incident Alzheimer's disease and cognitive decline in older persons. Sleep. 2013;36(7):1027–32. https://doi.org/10.5665/sleep.2802.
11. Naumann A, Daum I. Narcolepsy: pathophysiology and neuropsychological changes. Behav Neurol. 2003;14(3–4):89–98.
12. Henry GK, Satz P, Heilbronner RL. Evidence of a perceptual-encoding deficit in narcolepsy? Sleep. 1993;16(2):123–7.
13. Rogers AE, Rosenberg RS. Tests of memory in narcoleptics. Sleep. 1990;13(1):42–52.
14. Hood B, Bruck D. Metamemory in narcolepsy. J Sleep Res. 1997;6(3):205–10.
15. Stepanski EJ, Markey JJ, Zorick FJ, Roth T. Psychometric profiles of patient populations with excessive daytime sleepiness. Henry Ford Hosp Med J. 1990;38(4):219–22.
16. Aloia MS, Ilniczky N, Di Dio P, Perlis ML, Greenblatt DW, Giles DE. Neuropsychological changes and treatment compliance in older adults with sleep apnea. J Psychosom Res. 2003;54(1):71–6.
17. Bédard MA, Montplaisir J, Richer F, Rouleau I, Malo J. Obstructive sleep apnea syndrome: pathogenesis of neuropsychological deficits. J Clin Exp Neuropsychol. 1991;13(6):950–64. https://doi.org/10.1080/01688639108405110.
18. Valencia-Flores M, Bliwise DL, Guilleminault C, Cilveti R, Clerk A. Cognitive function in patients with sleep apnea after acute nocturnal nasal continuous positive airway pressure (CPAP) treatment: sleepiness and hypoxemia effects. J Clin Exp Neuropsychol. 1996;18(2):197–210. https://doi.org/10.1080/01688639608408275.
19. Beebe DW, Wells CT, Jeffries J, Chini B, Kalra M, Amin R. Neuropsychological effects of pediatric obstructive sleep apnea. J Int Neuropsychol Soc. 2004;10(7):962–75.

20. Beebe DW. Neurobehavioral effects of childhood sleep-disordered breathing (SDB): a comprehensive review. Sleep. 2006;29(9):1115–34.
21. Biggs SN, Vlahnadonis A, Anderson V, Bourke R, Nixon GM, Davey MJ, Home RS. Long-term changes in neurocognition and behavior following treatment of sleep disordered breathing in school-aged children. Sleep. 2014;37(1):77–84. https://doi.org/10.5665/sleep.3312.
22. Friedmann BC, Hendeles-Amitai A, Kozminsky E, Leiberman A, Friger M, Tarasiuk A, Tal A. Adenotonsillectomy improves neurocognitive function in children with obstructive sleep apnea syndrome. Sleep. 2003;26(8):999–1005.
23. Taylor HG, Bowen SR, Beebe DW, Hodges E, Amin R, Arens R, Chervin RD, Garetz SL, Katz ES, Moore RH, Morales KH, Muzumdar H, Paruthi S, Rosen CL, Sadhwani A, Thomas NH, Ware J, Marcus CL, Ellenberg SS, Redline S, Giordani B. Cognitive effects of adenotonsillectomy for obstructive sleep apnea. Pediatrics. 2016;138(2). https://doi.org/10.1542/peds.2015-4458.
24. Garetz SL. Behavior, cognition, and quality of life after adenotonsillectomy for pediatric sleep disordered breathing: summary of the literature. Otolaryngol Head Neck Surg. 2008;138(1 Suppl):S19–26. https://doi.org/10.1016/j.otohns.2007.06.738.
25. Smedje H, Broman JE, Hetta J. Associations between disturbed sleep and behavioural difficulties in 635 children aged six to eight years: a study based on parent perceptions. Eur Child Adolesc Psychiatry. 2001;10(1):1–9.
26. Naegele B, Thouvard V, Pepin JL, Levy P, Bonnet C, Perret JE, Pellat J, Feuerstein C. Deficits of cognitive executive functions in patients with sleep apnea syndrome. Sleep. 1995;18(1):43–52.
27. Galbiati A, Verga L, Giora E, Zucconi M, Ferini-Strambi L. The risk of neurodegeneration in REM sleep behavior disorder: a systematic review and meta-analysis of longitudinal studies. Sleep Med Rev. 2019;43:37–46. https://doi.org/10.1016/j.smrv.2018.09.008.
28. Yaffe K, Nasrallah I, Hoang TD, Lauderdale DS, Knutson KL, Carnethon MR, Launer LJ, Lewis CE, Sidney S. Sleep duration and white matter quality in middle-aged adults. Sleep. 2016;39(9):1743–7. https://doi.org/10.5665/sleep.6104.
29. Ooms S, Overeem S, Besse K, Rikkert MO, Verbeek M, Claassen JA. Effect of 1 night of total sleep deprivation on cerebrospinal fluid beta-amyloid 42 in healthy middle-aged men: a randomized clinical trial. JAMA Neurol. 2014;71(8):971–7. https://doi.org/10.1001/jamaneurol.2014.1173.
30. Dutil C, Walsh JJ, Featherstone RB, Gunnell KE, Tremblay MS, Gruber R, Weiss SK, Cote KA, Sampson M, Chaput J. Influence of sleep on developing brain functions and structures in children and adolescents: a systematic review. Sleep Med Rev. 2018;42:184–201. https://doi.org/10.1016/j.smrv.2018.08.003.

Telesleep Medicine

19

Amir Sharafkhaneh, Shahram Moghtader,
Bita Farhadpour, Supriya Singh, and Mary Rose

Introduction

Access to care is provided traditionally through face-to-face patient-provider inter-actions. The limitations of the current model of delivering medical care include timely access to a subspecialist, need for travel to long distances, and the issue of space for clinical care and related expenses. The new model of care overcomes these limitations through the use of new and upcoming telecommunication technologies.

Telehealth broadly is defined as access to health-care providers and services any-where and at any time. Telehealth can be provided in real-time (synchronous) or as stored and forward (asynchronous) services [1]. Telehealth covers a variety of ser-vices including inpatient and outpatient care, population health, home health care, second medical opinion, provider-to-provider consultation, group/individual educa-tion and counseling, group/individual physical rehabilitation, group/individual anti-addiction counseling and care, diagnostic interpretative services, and quality control of various medical services [2].

Sleep disorder diagnosis and management can be a perfect field for the applica-tion of telehealth. The diagnosis of sleep disorders heavily relies on the history and use of various questionnaires. The physician examination is mostly visual or auscul-tation rather than relying on palpation. Further, the relevant diagnostic tests are entirely in digital format and, thus, easily transferrable. Various device therapy options for sleep apnea provide remote access to the use of data. Interesting,

A. Sharafkhaneh (✉) · S. Moghtader · S. Singh
Michael E. DeBakey VA Medical Center, Department of Medicine, Houston, TX, USA
e-mail: amirs@bcm.edu

B. Farhadpour
Dignity Health, Houston, TX, USA

M. Rose
Baylor College of Medicine, Department of Medicine, Houston, TX, USA

© Springer Nature Switzerland AG 2021
I. S. Khawaja, T. D. Hurwitz (eds.), *Sleep Disorders in Selected Psychiatric Settings*, https://doi.org/10.1007/978-3-030-59309-4_19

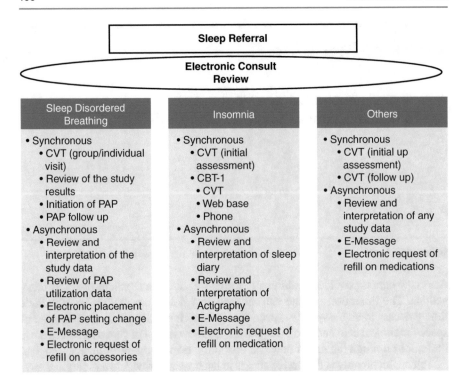

Fig. 19.1 Spectrum of sleep services that can be provided using telemedicine

telehealth, including tele-education and training, has been used to start sleep centers in countries that the knowledge in sleep medicine is scarce and thus is underserved. Various sleep disorder centers, including ours, started experimenting, implementing, and delivering initial and follow-up care of patients with sleep disorders through the use of telehealth technologies. In this chapter, we refer to telehealth for sleep disorders as telesleep (TS) [3, 4]. Figure 19.1 shows spectrum of sleep services that can be provided using telemedicine.

Telemedicine and Sleep-Disordered Breathing (SDB)

Application of Telemedicine for Diagnosis of SDB

The growth of telemedicine services overall has increased significantly in recent years. Many institutions and professional societies have incorporated or promoted telemedicine, including TS, as a viable option to one-on-one visits with the providers to improve access to quality primary and specialist care [5–7].

In sleep medicine, there is a history of successful use of telemedicine in the diagnosis of sleep disorders, including the diagnosis of sleep-disordered breathing. Studies done in recent years have shown the acceptance of TS and patient satisfaction in the diagnosis and management of sleep apnea, including teleconsultations [7].

The American Telemedicine Association Guidelines propose the technical requirements for TS's successful implementation [8]. These guidelines include the bandwidth, resolution, and software requirements as well as the diagnostic equipment, safety, and privacy needs for telehealth use.

Diagnostic testing is needed to be performed based on the standards as set by the American Academy of Sleep Medicine (AASM). Home Sleep Test (HST), also called Home Sleep Apnea Test (HSAT) equipment, is also to be used according to the current standards of care. Additionally, interpretation of sleep studies should be in accordance with the AASM manual for scoring. Sleep specialists may, however, make patient-specific recommendations along with these interpretations to improve patient-specific managements.

Our team has been using TS for diagnosis of sleep apnea for close to a decade. In our model, after reviewing the consult by a sleep specialist, patients with high risk for sleep apnea are scheduled to a group class. The HSAT devices are initialized for each specific patient and are shipped to the remote site. For each diagnostic session, one or more sites may join through video classes. At the beginning of each session, a sleep expert will review relevant issues related to sleep apnea, risk factors, and related adverse clinical outcomes. The expert then provides general instructions about preparation for testing and allows time for questions and answers. Subsequently, in our center, a respiratory therapist familiar with the device will train the patients on how to set the device on them for the testing. After the testing, the devices are returned either personally to the remote center or mailed in a padded envelope to the sleep center. The HSAT data is downloaded to the network and is reviewed and interpreted by a sleep expert. After being posted in the electronic medical record, the results relayed to patients by a respiratory therapist with a phone call. In summary, in our model of TS for diagnosis of SDB, we use both synchronous and asynchronous telehealth services.

Application of Telemedicine for Management of SDB

Positive airway pressure is the recommended treatment for obstructive sleep apnea. The American Academy of Sleep Medicine established a comprehensive document outlining titration with PAP during an attended sleep study [9]. Newer PAP technologies provide various methods of monitoring changes in respiratory flow and snoring and adjust the pressure using various algorithms [10]. The automatic PAP or APAP can provide details of various types of respiratory events nightly and in a summary format.

Further, PAP manufacturers provide the remote capability to monitor use and efficacy data. APAP allows for the initiation and adjustment of PAP pressure without a need for attended overnight titration in a large number of cases. Current contraindications for the use of automatic PAP include morbid obesity, advanced cardiac and respiratory disorders, central sleep apnea, advanced neurological disorders, and chronic use of medications that cause central respiratory events like narcotics [10, 11].

TS and Initiation of PAP Treatment

APAP and remote monitoring technologies fit very well in the TS model of delivering sleep services. In our institute, after diagnosis of SDB, a sleep expert reviews the electronic medical record for contraindications of APAP use. If none exists, patients are scheduled in a group class [10]. Other models may use a single provider-patient video interface due to insurance or confidentiality restrictions. The group class is conducted using video capabilities. Simultaneously, many of our community-based outpatient clinics (CBOC) connect and participate in the therapeutic group clinic. During this clinic, a sleep expert provides education on SDB, PAP and its use, and interfaces. An experienced respiratory therapist trains the patients on how to operate the device. An onsite health-care provider with prior training and experience on PAP interfaces fits the patients with proper interfaces. The patients return in a week with the SD card so that a sleep expert can review the use and efficacy data, and proper adjustment can be made to the pressure range. In a more recent model in our center, trained respiratory therapists, using the PAP remote data monitoring capabilities, review the utilization and efficacy data after a week of use and discuss the information with a sleep physician. The therapist, subsequently, communicates the findings and needed changes over the phone or using VA-specific smartphone applications with the patients. Various models of SDB diagnosis exist that mostly depends on practice setting, third-party payers' regulations, and privacy-related restrictions [3, 4].

TS and Follow-Up of PAP Treatment

PAP utilization is a major issue in treatment of SDB [12–14]. Therefore, close follow-up of SDB patients is crucial in optimal management of SDB. Although a set pressure may be efficacious in reducing respiratory events to a normal range, lack of adequate use makes PAP ineffective in producing favorable clinical outcomes. TS provides a methodology to more conveniently following these patients. Originally, our team of trained respiratory therapists would receive SD cards with related data through the mail, review the data with a sleep physician, call the patient to find out about their potential problems, and make an adjustment on pressure settings is needed. More recently, the patients are followed through an already-established and secure database. The convenience and ease of access to the data may improve utilization and, thus, the outcome. However, definitive data on the superiority of TS in improving utilization is pending more research. For a more detail review of TS and PAP follow-up, readers are referred to an excellent review by Dennis Hwang [15].

Methods to enhance diagnostic and clinical decision-making in TS include [1]:

1. Patient presenters are persons who facilitate the communication between the patient at the originating location and the sleep provider at the distant site. Their responsibilities include moving the patient in front of the camera or adjusting the audiovisual system for more accuracy in diagnosis and physical exam as well as clarification of certain communications between the patients and the provider.

2. Locally available sleep providers such as nurse practitioners or physician assistants may also be utilized for diagnostic accuracy. The hiring and training of these specialized assistants are to be done based on the local resources and guidelines.
3. Questionnaires and other tools such as the Epworth Sleepiness Scale need to be readily available to the TS providers.
4. Positive Airway Pressure (PAP) Download information also needs to be available to the TS clinicians based on the device manufacturers' guidelines to improve the clinician's diagnostic accuracy. Methods to enhance sleep provider's access to this information should be developed [16].
5. Additional diagnostic testing such as spirometry, echocardiography, electrocardiography, and home oximetry results are also needed to be available to the sleep providers in certain situations to improve diagnostic accuracy.
6. The utilization of peripheral devices such as electronic stethoscopes for heart and lung examinations also needs to be available to the providers in a particular situation when clinically warranted.
7. The roles of physicians, physician assistants, respiratory therapists, sleep technologists, nurse practitioners, licensed practical nurses, registered nurses, and medical office assistants and others need to be clarified in the process of TS practice, and contingency plans should also be in place in certain situations such as equipment failure or in case of an emergency.

Telemedicine and Behavioral Sleep Medicine (Mary Rose)

Many providers consider insomnia to be synonymous with behavioral sleep medicine. However, there is a gamut of behavioral sleep issues in which we might make an impact. Developing a comprehensive assessment of the psychological factors which influence sleep has come increasingly into the forefront. TS holds the promise not only of assessment and treatment but of monitoring to ensure continued treatment and troubleshooting of the myriad of factors that can negatively impact numerous sleep disorders. The complications of telemedicine are relatively well understood; technology may impede representation of medical conditions related to skin discoloration (leading to missed conditions such as jaundice and iron deficiency), olfaction which is sometimes an indicator of conditions such as infection, or other conditions. Identification of conditions which a practitioner might otherwise become aware of visually serendipitously may also be missed. However, assessments of *psychological* factors which influence the course of a sleep disorder are less vulnerable to these shortcomings. TS for psychologically impacted sleep disorders may target a range of sleep complaints and broaden access to care.

In all areas of sleep, behavioral medicine is a necessary tool in comprehensively understanding any sleep disorder, as well as issues that may block adherence to treatment(s).

Telemedicine (TM) and telehealth (TH) have been a rapidly expanding area of health care [17]. For this paper, TM will be used to encompass telehealth and to discuss TS services overall. It is difficult to differentiate the concepts of telemedicine and telehealth. Regarding TS, not only are the more concretely defined aspects of physical medicine critical, but behavioral medicine as well. Not only is untreated OSA associated with multiple medical severe comorbidities, but it is almost always well managed via CPAP, with few side effects. Though adherence issues are generally associated with issues such as claustrophobia from the mask [18], patients often develop higher tolerance and commitment to usage when their results have been reviewed with them; they know that PAP is a likely treatment option before being evaluated and that it often takes some troubleshooting to find the ideal mask. For patients in more remote areas, telehealth provides greater assurance that patients receive this critical information and can troubleshoot as they adapt to PAP use.

In recent years, computerized cognitive-behavioral therapy (CCBT) has rapidly expanded to offer structured CBT programs via Internet-based or mHealth (mobile health apps). These are generally grounded in the basic principles of CBT, but are self-driven [19, 20]. These programs appear to have mild to moderate benefit on insomnia, per a recent meta-analysis [21], and to be overall moderately useable [22]. Studies involving trained providers, however, indicate that TS delivery of CBT is effective for both depression and insomnia [23, 24]. Contrary to Internet programs in which no provider is involved, TS is clinician-driven TM care. Availability of remote care has been invaluable in several incidences: environment with high volume patient care needs, those in which patient travel is restricted due to excessive distances, medical conditions limiting travel ability, and mental health issues. For many facilities, more than one of these conditions exist; thus, TM allows access to care which would likely be significantly delayed or prevented where TM is not available. TM additionally frees up clinic space and promotes more regular follow-up and access to care. Patients can be roomed by nursing at a remote center, which reduces clinician downtime in rooming patients locally, and smaller centers local to patients are likely to offer better parking options and fewer obstacles, which may delay patient access to the clinic itself. Remote TM-based CBT-I has been proven as effective as face-to-face standard of care in multiple studies. On one study, web-based delivery from home was compared with telehealth-based delivery from a nearby clinic [25]. Both interventions contained identical content: psycho-education, sleep hygiene, stimulus control instruction, sleep restriction treatment, relaxation training, cognitive therapy, mindfulness meditation, and medication-tapering assistance. They found that though both delivery methods produced equivalent changes in the severity of insomnia, web-based delivery was associated with homework, while telehealth was associated with higher attendance [25, 26].

Utilizing nurse providers in a study comparing usual care vs TM, patients treated under a TM protocol had comparable benefits to those with direct face-to-face usual care [26]. Both treatment groups indicated CPAP usage hours (>4 h/day) and no change in PAP usage at the end of the habituation. Both groups were equally satisfied with their treatment. At 1-year follow-up, CPAP use and residual AHI were excellent in both groups. However, a notable difference was found in the time requirement on the providers, with the TM group being associated with less time requirement [26]. Parikh et al. conducted a large-scale study that suggested no difference between those with in-person follow-up and those being seen via telemedicine follow-up with regard to either satisfaction with care or PAP usage [7]. Another study, though requiring more extensive telephone follow-up and remote monitoring than the standard of care, likewise showed better results from TM than with standard of care in PAP adherence [27].

TM is widely used within the Veteran's Administration Hospitals. Of the 127 VAMC sleep centers surveyed, 40 reported use of TM in their clinical practice.

There are multiple areas in which TM can be easily used to aid in the evaluation of most sleep disorders. The most common uses to date have included: orientation and demonstration for diagnostic testing or obstructive sleep apnea, individual sleep evaluations, and follow-up on disorders such as obstructive sleep apnea (OSA), REM behavior disorder (RBD), narcolepsy, insomnia, and circadian rhythm disorder. The most productive use of TM that we have found is in the group orientation to OSA evaluation and treatment of OSA. OSA is a common and serious disorder that is relatively easily screened and easily treated via positive airway pressure (PAP). With the increase in obesity in the USA, an increase in OSA is likely to continue rising. As OSA is associated with high morbidity and negatively impedes other medical conditions such as HTN, obesity, stroke, diabetes, and mood disorders, evaluation and treatment can provide a significant improvement to health-related quality of life and overall quality of life.

Insomnia, with little debate, presents as the most challenging of sleep disorders. This is related to multiple factors. The causes of insomnia are multifold and rarely perpetuated solely by a medical condition such as hyperthyroidism. Other sleep disorders such as periodic limb movement disorder and OSA [28] can be provocateurs of insomnia. However, other common causes include substance use, PTSD, anxiety, depression, and irregular work schedules. PTSD, though certainly not unique to veterans, is more prevalent than in non-veterans [29]. Those presenting with insomnia as a primary sleep complaint have often had multiple previous and sometimes concurrent treatments for insomnia. In the VA system, patients are often being treated in mental health pharmacologically for other comorbid mental health issues and insomnia.

A comprehensive sleep questionnaire and other materials can be provided to patients at the origination site to complete or mailed, then faxed back, or securely sent to the provider for review. This expedites time for the patient and the clinician. A well-structured sleep questionnaire provides a comprehensive description of sleep symptoms, which facilitates ease of diagnosis and treatment planning. An additional benefit is that it often illuminates for the patient the range of type of symptoms they are experiencing and aids in their collaboration during the assessment.

We have found that some patients being treated long-term for behavioral sleep issues such as insomnia and PAP adherence request occasional face-to-face interaction with providers, which is usually cited as a desire for acquiring at least one face-to-face personal contact with the provider.

Telemedicine has rapidly improved access to care for patients from remote areas to receive the care they would otherwise be unlikely to obtain. Additionally, it allows patients to tap into a broader range of services and service providers.

Technical Aspects of Telemedicine

Figure 19.2 depicts various aspects of establishing a telemedicine program. The components include medical, technical, financial, legal, and marketing aspects. A fundamental issue is to have champions from health-care providers who are willing to identify the needs that may benefit from telemedicine. For example, in our institute, timely access to medical care for veterans is the number one priority. The practitioners also help to critically review the existing literature and develop or adapt models of care for the practice setting. A strong information technology expertise is of utmost importance to assure that the required infrastructure exists for the implementation of telemedicine services. Further, identifying suitable hardware and software for delivering the care relies on not only the practitioners and IT teams but also the compliance team to ensure that privacy issues are addressed adequately. Last but not least is sorting out the billing and codes that can be used [1].

The primary activity of starting a telemedicine program is to gather the required team (Fig. 19.2). In our institute, the telemedicine team evaluated how the sleep center provides current face-to-face services and how sleep providers perceive TS will align with their current processes. We identified physician champions to be responsible for the clinical aspects of TS and operation champions to collaborate with the physician champions to design and manage the TS program. Additionally, we defined the role and expectations of each TS clinic staff. The telemedicine team also assured that licensing and credentialing requirements are met; developed policy

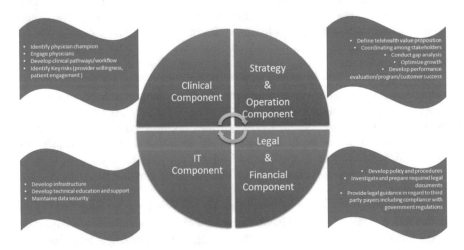

Fig. 19.2 Various components and stakeholders that should be considered when starting a telemedicine program

and procedure, business agreement, telehealth-related consent form, and workflow; defined the reimbursement; and created marketing and communication strategies.

In stark contrast with the traditional health-care delivery model of in-person visits, telemedicine connects two different sites: a distant site where practitioners provide the care and originating site with patients receiving the care. The telemedicine team is in charge of identifying and preparing both types of sites to implement telemedicine.

Preparing the sites includes but is not limited to identifying practitioners and staff, developing the needed infrastructure, finalizing agreements, and providing training. Before the start of any telemedicine program, a soft run of the program at a minimal scale is warranted to identify any problems before going live.

Sleep services using telemedicine technology provide a reliable alternative to the traditional model of medical care and may improve access to care, particularly in places that subspecialized sleep care is not readily available. As telemedicine grows, its regulatory, technical, and financial aspects grow too. Forming a telemedicine committee and developing needed documents is a priority before starting any telesleep services.

References

1. Singh J, Badr MS, Diebert W, et al. American Academy of Sleep Medicine (AASM) position paper for the use of telemedicine for the diagnosis and treatment of sleep disorders. J Clin Sleep Med. 2015;11(10):1187–98.
2. Kvedar J, Coye MJ, Everett W. Connected health: a review of technologies and strategies to improve patient care with telemedicine and telehealth. Health Aff (Millwood). 2014;33(2):194–9.
3. Verbraecken J. Telemedicine applications in sleep disordered breathing: thinking out of the box. Sleep Med Clin. 2016;11(4):445–59.
4. Bruyneel M. Technical developments and clinical use of telemedicine in sleep medicine. J Clin Med. 2016;5(12):116.
5. Wechsler LR, Tsao JW, Levine SR, et al. Teleneurology applications: report of the Telemedicine Work Group of the American Academy of Neurology. Neurology. 2013;80(7):670–6.
6. Lilly CM, Zubrow MT, Kempner KM, et al. Critical care telemedicine: evolution and state of the art. Crit Care Med. 2014;42(11):2429–36.
7. Parikh R, Touvelle MN, Wang H, Zallek SN. Sleep telemedicine: patient satisfaction and treatment adherence. Telemed J E Health. 2011;17(8):609–14.
8. Gough F, Budhrani S, Cohn E, et al. ATA practice guidelines for live, on-demand primary and urgent care. Telemed J E Health. 2015;21(3):233–41.
9. Kushida CA, Chediak A, Berry RB, et al. Clinical guidelines for the manual titration of positive airway pressure in patients with obstructive sleep apnea. J Clin Sleep Med. 2008;4(2):157–71.
10. Hirshkowitz M, Sharafkhaneh A. A telemedicine program for diagnosis and management of sleep-disordered breathing: the fast-track for sleep apnea tele-sleep program. Semin Respir Crit Care Med. 2014;35(5):560–70.
11. Littner M, Hirshkowitz M, Davila D, et al. Practice parameters for the use of auto-titrating continuous positive airway pressure devices for titrating pressures and treating adult patients with obstructive sleep apnea syndrome. An American Academy of Sleep Medicine report. Sleep. 2002;25(2):143–7.

12. Taylor Y, Eliasson A, Andrada T, Kristo D, Howard R. The role of telemedicine in CPAP compliance for patients with obstructive sleep apnea syndrome. Sleep Breath. 2006;10(3):132–8.
13. Yetkin O, Kunter E, Gunen H. CPAP compliance in patients with obstructive sleep apnea syndrome. Sleep Breath. 2008;12(4):365–7.
14. Stepnowsky CJ Jr, Marler MR, Ancoli-Israel S. Determinants of nasal CPAP compliance. Sleep Med. 2002;3(3):239–47.
15. Hwang D. Monitoring progress and adherence with positive airway pressure therapy for obstructive sleep apnea: the roles of telemedicine and mobile health applications. Sleep Med Clin. 2016;11(2):161–71.
16. Schwab RJ, Badr SM, Epstein LJ, et al. An official American Thoracic Society statement: continuous positive airway pressure adherence tracking systems. The optimal monitoring strategies and outcome measures in adults. Am J Respir Crit Care Med. 2013;188(5):613–20.
17. Global telemedicine market size from 2015 to 2021 (in billion US dollars)*. Global telemedicine market size from 2015 to 2021 (in billion US dollars)* Web site. https://www.statista.com/statistics/671374/global-telemedicine-market-size/. Published 2019. Updated 4/23/19. Accessed.
18. Edmonds JC, Yang H, King TS, Sawyer DA, Rizzo A, Sawyer AM. Claustrophobic tendencies and continuous positive airway pressure therapy non-adherence in adults with obstructive sleep apnea. Heart Lung. 2015;44(2):100–6.
19. Chan C, West S, Glozier N. Commencing, and persisting with a web-based cognitive behavioral intervention for insomnia: a qualitative study of treatment completers. J Med Internet Res. 2017;19(2):e37.
20. Thorndike FP, Ritterband LM, Gonder-Frederick LA, Lord HR, Ingersoll KS, Morin CM. A randomized controlled trial of an internet intervention for adults with insomnia: effects on comorbid psychological and fatigue symptoms. J Clin Psychol. 2013;69(10):1078–93.
21. Cheng SK, Dizon J. Computerised cognitive behavioural therapy for insomnia: a systematic review and meta-analysis. Psychother Psychosom. 2012;81(4):206–16.
22. Yu JS, Kuhn E, Miller KE, Taylor K. Smartphone apps for insomnia: examining existing apps' usability and adherence to evidence-based principles for insomnia management. Transl Behav Med. 2019;9(1):110–9.
23. Lichstein KL, Scogin F, Thomas SJ, DiNapoli EA, Dillon HR, McFadden A. Telehealth cognitive behavior therapy for co-occurring insomnia and depression symptoms in older adults. J Clin Psychol. 2013;69(10):1056–65.
24. Scogin F, Lichstein K, DiNapoli EA, et al. Effects of integrated telehealth-delivered cognitive-behavioral therapy for depression and insomnia in rural older adults. J Psychother Integr. 2018;28(3):292–309.
25. Holmqvist M, Vincent N, Walsh K. Web- vs. telehealth-based delivery of cognitive-behavioral therapy for insomnia: a randomized controlled trial. Sleep Med. 2014;15(2):187–95.
26. Anttalainen U, Melkko S, Hakko S, Laitinen T, Saaresranta T. Telemonitoring of CPAP therapy may save nursing time. Sleep Breath. 2016;20(4):1209–15.
27. Fox N, Hirsch-Allen AJ, Goodfellow E, et al. The impact of a telemedicine monitoring system on positive airway pressure adherence in patients with obstructive sleep apnea: a randomized controlled trial. Sleep. 2012;35(4):477–81.
28. Cronlein T, Geisler P, Langguth B, et al. Polysomnography reveals unexpectedly high rates of organic sleep disorders in patients with prediagnosed primary insomnia. Sleep Breath. 2012;16(4):1097–103.
29. Smith SM, Goldstein RB, Grant BF. The association between post-traumatic stress disorder and lifetime DSM-5 psychiatric disorders among veterans: data from the National Epidemiologic Survey on Alcohol and Related Conditions-III (NESARC-III). J Psychiatr Res. 2016;82:16–22.

Index

© Springer Nature Switzerland AG 2021
I. S. Khawaja, T. D. Hurwitz (eds.), *Sleep Disorders in Selected
Psychiatric Settings*, https://doi.org/10.1007/978-3-030-59309-4

Printed in the United States
by Baker & Taylor Publisher Services